Narjes ABID
Soumaya DEBICHE

Etiological profile of spontaneous pneumothorax in 206 cases

Narjes ABID
Soumaya DEBICHE

Etiological profile of spontaneous pneumothorax in 206 cases

ScienciaScripts

Imprint
Any brand names and product names mentioned in this book are subject to trademark, brand or patent protection and are trademarks or registered trademarks of their respective holders. The use of brand names, product names, common names, trade names, product descriptions etc. even without a particular marking in this work is in no way to be construed to mean that such names may be regarded as unrestricted in respect of trademark and brand protection legislation and could thus be used by anyone.

Cover image: www.ingimage.com

This book is a translation from the original published under ISBN 978-620-6-72316-5.

Publisher:
Sciencia Scripts
is a trademark of
Dodo Books Indian Ocean Ltd. and OmniScriptum S.R.L publishing group

120 High Road, East Finchley, London, N2 9ED, United Kingdom
Str. Armeneasca 28/1, office 1, Chisinau MD-2012, Republic of Moldova, Europe
Managing Directors: Ieva Konstantinova, Victoria Ursu
info@omniscriptum.com

Printed at: see last page
ISBN: 978-620-8-38250-6

Table of contents

Table of contents **1**

I NTRODUCTION **5**

METHODS **7**

1. *Type and duration of study* *8*
2. *Inclusion criteria* *8*
3. *Non-inclusion criteria* *8*
4. *Exclusion criteria* *8*
5. *Data collection* *8*

5.1. Characteristics of patients 8

5.2. Characteristics of pneumothorax 9

5.3. Etiological diagnosis of spontaneous pneumothorax 11

5.3.1. Etiological assessment 11

5.3.2. Etiologies of spontaneous pneumothorax 12

5.4. Therapeutic management of pneumothorax : 12

5.4.1. Conservative treatment 12

5.4.2. Pleural evacuation 12

5.4.3. Medical or surgical pleurodesis. 12

5.5. Evolution 13

6. *Statistical analysis :* *14*

6.1. Descriptive study 14

6.2. Analytical study 14

6.3. Bibliographic research 14

6.4. Ethical considerations 14

RESULTS **15**

1. *Descriptive study* *16*

1.1. Patient characteristics 16

1.1.1. Socio-demographic characteristics 16

1.1.1.1. Age 16

1.1.1.2. Type 16

1.1.1.3. Habits 17

1.1.1.3.1. Smoking 17

1.1.1.3.2. Ethylism 17

1.1.1.3.3. Drug use 17

1.1.2. Comorbidities 17

1.1.2.1. Respiratory comorbidities 17

1.1.2.2. Extra-respiratory comorbidities 18

1.1.3. Anthropometric data 18

1.2. Characteristics of pneumothorax 18

1.2.1. Number of pneumothorax episodes 18

1.2.2. Consultation period 19

1.2.3. Circumstances of discovery 19

1.2.4. Clinical tolerance of pneumothorax 19

1.3. Radiological data 19

1.3.1. Radiological characteristics of pneumothorax 19

1.3.2. Chest CT scan 20

1.4. Etiological diagnosis of pneumothorax 23

1.4.1. Contribution of CT scans to etiological assessment 24

1.4.2. Etiologies of PSS 29

1.5. Therapeutic management 30

1.5.1. Conservative treatment 30

1.5.2. Pleural evacuation 31

1.5.3. Medical pleurodesis 31

1.6. Long-term trends 32

2. *Analytical study* *32*

2.1. Socio-demographic characteristics 32

2.1.1. Age 32

2.1.2. Type 33

2.1.3. Smoking 33

2.1.4. Anthropometric data 33

2.2. Clinical data 33

2.3. Radiological data 33

2.3.1. Thoracic CT scan indications according to PS etiology (Figure 19) . 34

2.3.2. Description of scan anomalies 34

1.1. Therapeutic data (Figure 21) 35

1.2. Scalable data 36

1.3. Summary and comparison between PSP and PSS 37

D ISCUSSION **39**

C ONCLUSIONS **52**

REF RENC ES **57**

APPENDICES **64**

List of abbreviations

ACCP: American College of Chest Physicians

BTS: British thoracic society

COPD: Chronic obstructive pulmonary disease

CHU: Centre Hospitalo-Universitaire

ERS: European Respiratory Society

VAS: Visual Analog Scale

BMI: Body Mass Index

PS: Spontaneous pneumothorax

PSP: Primary spontaneous pneumothorax

PSS: Secondary spontaneous pneumothorax

PA: Package-years

PAS: Systolic blood pressure

DIP: Diffuse Infiltrative Pneumopathy

SBP: Belgian Respiratory Society

SPSS: Statistical Package for Social Science

CT: computed tomography

TSVA: video-assisted thoracoscopy

I NTRODUCTION

Spontaneous pneumothorax (SP) is defined as the presence of a gaseous effusion in the pleural cavity due to the spontaneous irruption of air between the parietal and visceral pleura. It may be primary (primary spontaneous pneumothorax: PSP), affecting patients free of any respiratory pathology, or secondary (secondary spontaneous pneumothorax: PSS), when it complicates an underlying pulmonary pathology. Differentiation between these two entities is based on clinical and standard chest X-ray data. However, this distinction is becoming increasingly blurred, given that smoking is the main risk factor for both primary and secondary HP, and that many parenchymal lesions may be missed on the standard chest X-ray and can only be detected on chest CT. However, this examination is not systematically performed in the event of a first episode of PS, and its role is not yet well codified. [1, 2].

Recurrence is the main evolutionary risk of PS [3,4]. However, prevention of recurrence from the very first episode is not systematic, given the current lack of any reliable indicator for predicting the risk of recurrence in a particular patient. Numerous clinical and radiological parameters have been studied, but little is known about the role of CT scans in this indication. [5].

We thus carried out a prospective study, the main aim of which was to determine the etiological profile of PS treated at the Pneumology Department of the Mohamed Taher Mâamouri University Hospital Centre (CHU) in Nabeul, and to identify the role of chest CT in the etiological investigation of this condition. The secondary aim of our study was to determine the contribution of cross-sectional imaging in its therapeutic management.

METHODS

1. Type and duration of study

- This is a prospective study involving all patients hospitalized for PS at the pneumology department of CHU Mohamed Taher Mâamouri in Nabeul between August 2013 and December 2019.

2. Inclusion criteria

- Age 16 and over
- First episode or recurrence of a PS
- Minimum follow-up period: 1 year from hospital discharge date

3. Non-inclusion criteria

- Traumatic pneumothorax
- Iatrogenic pneumothorax

4. Exclusion criteria

- Patients lost to follow-up within 1 year of hospital discharge

5. Data collection

- A worksheet was drawn up to collect data from each patient (Appendix 1).
- Prospectively collected data included:

5.1. Characteristics of patients

The following were collected:

- Socio-demographic data: age, gender, origin, place of residence, occupation, level of education.
- Habits : smoking measured in pack-years (PY), cannabis or alcohol consumption.
- Comorbidities : respiratory and extra-respiratory. Pathologies predisposing to the development of PS were specified.
- The anthropometric parameters: weight, height and body mass index (BMI), morphotype (normal or lanky defined by a height/weight ratio ≥ 3 cm/kg).

5.2. Characteristics of pneumothorax

The SP characteristics collected included:

- Number of pneumothorax episodes: first episode or recurrence (homolateral or contralateral)
- Consultation time: defined as the time between the onset of symptoms and consultation.
- Circumstances of discovery: incidental finding, dyspnea, chest pain whose intensity has been assessed by the visual analog scale (VAS) and defined as mild for a VAS value <3, moderate for a value between 3 and 5 and severe for a value >5, dyspnea and ~~other~~.
- Clinical tolerance of pneumothorax :
  - Respiratory impact was judged on the presence of signs of acute respiratory failure (polypnoea defined as an increase in respiratory rate above 20 cycles/min, signs of respiratory struggle: intercostal, supra-sternal or supra-clavicular pulling, cyanosis).
  - Hemodynamic impact was judged by the presence of signs of acute circulatory failure defined as systolic blood pressure (SBP) <90 mm Hg or a drop in SBP of more than 30% from baseline in hypertensive patients or patients with habitually low blood pressure.

A pneumothorax was considered to be poorly tolerated if it had respiratory and/or hemodynamic repercussions.

- The radiological characteristics recorded from the chest X-ray taken at the time of diagnosis of PS for all patients :
  - ➢ The total or partial nature of the PS: according to the Belgian Society of Pneumology (SBP), a total pneumothorax is defined by complete dehiscence of the lung over the entire height of the chest wall, while a partial pneumothorax is defined by partial dehiscence. [6].
  - ➢ The size of the PS: a pneumothorax of great abundance is defined by an interpleural distance (distance measured on the frontal chest X-ray between the visceral pleura and the parietal pleura) at the hilum greater than or equal to two centimeters according to the criteria of the British Thoracic Society (BTS). [1] and greater than three centimetres measured at the lung apex according to the criteria of the American College of Chest Physicians (ACCP) [7].

- ➢ PS seat: right, left or bilateral.

- Chest X-ray abnormalities suggesting underlying parenchymal pathology: emphysema, bronchial syndrome or areolar opacities suggestive of bronchial dilatation, interstitial syndrome, intra-parenchymal round opacity, apical retractile opacity suggestive of tuberculosis sequelae, cavitary syndrome defined by the presence of intrapulmonary clarity surrounded by a wall of variable thickness from one millimeter to several centimeters. When this wall is thin, less than two millimeters, and regular, the image is said to be cystic [8].

- Chest computed tomography (CT) data included:
    - Indication for a CT scan as part of the initial workup: a chest CT scan was performed in accordance with the recommendations of the European Respiratory Society (ERS). [9]:
        - ✓ In case of diagnostic doubt, notably between a partial pneumothorax and an emphysema bulla
        - ✓ As part of the etiological assessment of PS, particularly in cases of doubt about an underlying respiratory pathology not supported by clinical and chest X-ray evidence
        - ✓ In the event of a suspected thoracic drainage complication
        - ✓ As part of the pre-operative assessment
    - Time taken to perform a chest CT scan in relation to the positive diagnosis of pneumothorax.
    - Signs in favor of pneumothorax repercussions or complications: deviation of mediastinal structures towards the contralateral side, associated homolateral liquid pleural effusion, atelectasis or ventilatory disturbance opposite the pneumothorax, pneumomediastinum, pleural flanges.
    - Parenchymal abnormalities potentially incriminating in the occurrence of pneumothorax or in favor of an underlying parenchymal pathology such as :
        - ✓ Blebs are thin-walled cystic airspaces less than one centimetre in diameter, contiguous with the pleural space [8].
        - ✓ Pulmonary emphysema is defined by abnormal dilatation of the airspaces beyond the terminal bronchiole, accompanied by destruction of the alveolar

partitions with no obvious associated fibrosis. It is classified as centrolobular when it mainly affects the proximal respiratory bronchioles and the alveoli located in the central part of the acinus, paraseptal when it selectively affects the alveolar partitions located in contact with the interlobular septa, and panlobular when it involves the airspaces of the acinus and the lobule as a whole. Bullous emphysema is the association of centro-lobular or paraseptal emphysema with bullae corresponding to areas of emphysema over a centimetre in diameter, sometimes surrounded by thin wall [8].

- ✓ Pulmonary emphysema was assessed qualitatively, without quantitative scoring of lesion extent.
- ✓ Nodule or excavated mass in contact with the pleura
- ✓ Cystic or cavitary image defined by a well-demarcated thin-walled aerated lesion free of internal anatomical structure or solid material [10].
- ✓ Diffuse infiltrative pneumonitis (DIP) with honeycomb images [8].
- ✓ Sequelae of tuberculosis: condensation or collapsed lung scarring with bronchial dilatation or residual cavity

- Chest CT scans were high-resolution for all patients, with volume acquisition (16 bars) extending from the pulmonary apexes to the lower pole of the liver.
- Parenchymal abnormalities detected by chest CT but not visualized by standard radiography are termed infra-radiological.

5.3. Etiological diagnosis of spontaneous pneumothorax

5.3.1. Etiological assessment

It was based on a number of parameters:

- Patient's age
- The notion of smoking. Heavy smoking is defined as consuming more than 20 cigarettes a day.
- Existence of a known respiratory pathology
- The existence of clinical or radiological signs on the chest X-ray suggesting pulmonary pathology

5.3.2. Etiologies of spontaneous pneumothorax

PS was classified as primary or secondary based on the BTS definition which considers as PSS any pneumothorax occurring in a patient over 50 years of age with a history of heavy smoking or in a patient who presents clinical signs or abnormalities on the standard chest radiograph made at the time of PS diagnosis, in favor of a pulmonary pathology [1]. In all other cases, the pneumothorax was considered primary (PSP).

The etiologies of SP have been clarified.

5.4. Therapeutic management of pneumothorax :

5.4.1. Conservative treatment

Conservative treatment consists of bed rest with high-concentration mask oxygen therapy at a flow rate of between 8 and 10 l/min.

5.4.2. Pleural evacuation

The pleural evacuation modalities were:

5.4.2.1. Needle exsufflation

Successful exsufflation is defined according to the BTS by an interpleural distance opposite the hilum of less than two centimetres after exsufflation, with improvement in dyspnoea in the case of large-abundance PSP, and by an interpleural distance of less than one centimetre after exsufflation, whereas it was between one and two centimetres before pleural evacuation in the case of small-abundance PSS. [1].

5.4.2.2. Chest drainage

Successful drainage, whether immediate (≤48 hours) or delayed (time in days), has been defined according to BTS by a return of the lung to the wall or an interpleural distance<2 cm [1].

5.4.3. Medical or surgical pleurodesis.

Pleurodesis, or pleural symphysis, is a process whereby the two pleural layers are joined together. It can be medical by injecting a sclerosing agent through the drain (the product used is talc slurry diluted in 20 cc of physiological serum injected in one go or povidone iodine combined with 10 cc of Xylocaine and 20 cc of physiological serum injected 3 days in a row) or surgical (mechanical by pleural abrasion and/or pleurectomy or chemical by injecting a sclerosing agent between the two pleural sheets intraoperatively).

Pleurodesis is indicated in cases of :

- Recurrent pneumothorax defined by the occurrence of a second PS homolateral or contralateral to the first episode.
- A persistent pneumothorax defined by the absence of return of the lung to the wall beyond 7 days of thoracic drainage [1].
- A two-way PS from the outset.
- Spontaneous hemopneumothorax
- A PS occurring in a patient working in a high-risk profession such as airline pilots.

Medical pleurodesis through the drain is reserved for cases where surgery is not possible due to a contraindication to general anaesthesia. In all other cases, surgical pleurodesis is performed. Intraoperative findings have been reported, as have the operative procedures associated with pleurodesis.

5.5. Evolution

Evolutionary data of the PS during hospitalization included:

- Complications of thoracic drainage
- Length of hospital stay

Patients are followed up after discharge by a lung specialist. The follow-up schedule included :

- First consultation on average 7 days after hospital discharge
- Followed by consultations at one month, three months and one year

Data collected during follow-up consultations included:

- Clinical data:
  - ✓ Assessment of chest pain using VAS
  - ✓ Physical examination data (respiratory rate, pulse oxygen saturation, blood pressure, heart rate)
  - ✓ The condition of the drainage or exsufflation scar
  - ✓ Smoking

- Radiological data
  - ✓ Lung wall or detached
  - ✓ Parenchymal anomalies
  - ✓ Chest CT scan data during follow-up

Recurrences were recorded along with their characteristics: time to onset, and whether they were homolateral or contralateral to the first episode.

6. Statistical analysis :

Data were entered and analyzed using SPSS (Statistical Package for Social Science) version 20 software.

6.1. Descriptive study

- ➢ Quantitative values are expressed as mean and standard deviation.
- ➢ Qualitative values were expressed in terms of frequency and number of employees.

6.2. Analytical study

For the statistical analysis and comparative study, the following tests were used:

- ➢ The STUDENT test for independent quantitative values.
- ➢ The KHI2 test for qualitative values.

The difference is considered statistically significant when p is less than 0.05.

6.3. Bibliographic research

We used the search engine: pubmed.ncbi.nlm.nih.gov and the following bibliographic search site: www.sciencedirect.com

6.4. Ethical considerations

We declare that we have no conflict of interest in this study and that medical confidentiality has been respected.

RESULTS

During the period of our study [August 2013 to December 2019], 206 cases of PS were recorded.

1. Descriptive study

1.1. Patient characteristics

1.1.1. Socio-demographic characteristics

1.1.1.1. Age

The mean age of our patients was 40±18 years, with extremes ranging from 16 to 87 years. Nearly half the patients (49%; n=101) were between 20 and 40 years of age. Sixty-five patients (31.6%) were over 50 years of age (Figure 1).

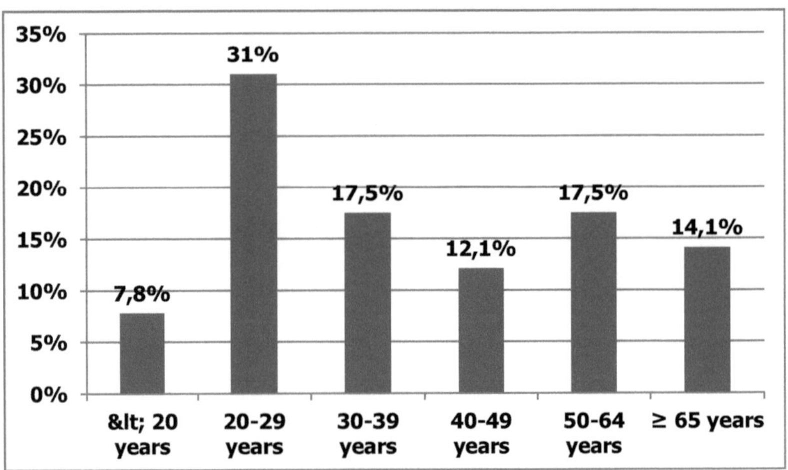

Figure 1Patient distribution by age group

1.1.1.2. Type

Our population was clearly male-dominated (201 men (97.6%) and 5 women (2.4%)) with a gender-ratio M/F of 40.2 (Figure 2).

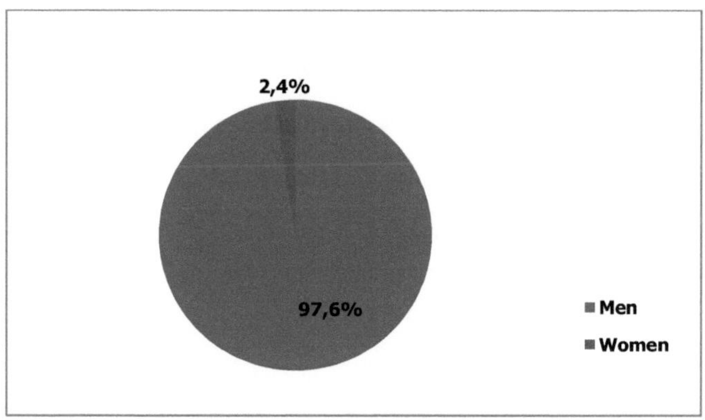

Figure 2Patient distribution by gender

1.1.1.3. Habits

1.1.1.3.1. Smoking

The majority of patients were smokers (183 patients; 88.8%). Average annual smoking was 27±22 BP [1- 120 BP]. Twenty-one patients were weaned from smoking at the time of diagnosis (10%).

1.1.1.3.2. Ethylism

Forty-seven patients (22.8%) were regular alcohol consumers.

1.1.1.3.3. Drug use

Cannabis use was reported by nine patients (4.3%).

1.1.2. Comorbidities

1.1.2.1. Respiratory comorbidities

Pulmonary pathology was already known at the time of PS diagnosis in 26.7% of our patients (n=55 cases). Pathologies predisposing to PS were noted in 51 patients (24.7%). They were represented by :

- Chronic obstructive pulmonary disease (COPD) in 36 patients (17.5%).
- Pulmonary tuberculosis in 12 patients (5.8%). It was active in three patients and cured with parenchymal sequelae in nine.
- Fibrosing PID in two patients (1%) (one case of idiopathic pulmonary fibrosis and one case of mediastino-pulmonary sarcoidosis).

- Primary pulmonary neoplasia in one patient.

Other respiratory comorbidities were represented by asthma in four patients (2%).

1.1.2.2. Extra-respiratory comorbidities

Extra-respiratory comorbidities were found in 30 patients (15%) and included :

- Cardiovascular diseases: hypertension (13 patients; 6.3%), rhythm disorders (three patients; 1.5%), coronary insufficiency (three patients; 1.5%), stroke (one patient; 0.5%) and peripheral arterial disease (one patient; 0.5%).
- Diabetes (six patients; 2.9%).
- Peptic ulcer disease (five patients; 2.4%).
- Extra thoracic neoplasia in two patients (1%) (one case of bladder carcinoma and one case of rectal tumour).

1.1.3. Anthropometric data

Forty-five patients (21.8%) had a lanky morphotype. The mean BMI was 21.03±3 kg/m^2 [15.02- 32.7 kg/m^2]. Most patients had a mean BMI of less than 25kg/m^2 (Figure 3).

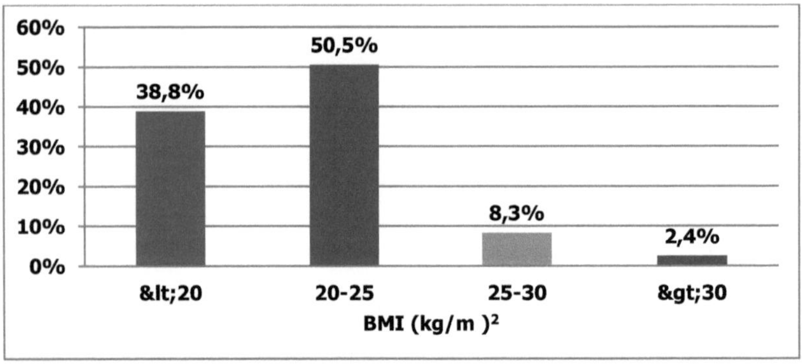

Figure 3 Distribution of patients by body mass index

1.2. Characteristics of pneumothorax

1.2.1. Number of pneumothorax episodes

Twenty patients (9%) had a history of PS (homolateral to the episode studied in 12 cases and contralateral to this episode in eight cases).

1.2.2. Consultation period

Two-thirds of patients (n=136; 66%) consulted us on the first day of symptom onset, with an average delay of 14 h [1 hour-24 hours]. In the other cases, the average consultation time was 4±3 days, with extremes ranging from 2 to 20 days.

1.2.3. Circumstances of discovery

Chest pain was the most frequent symptom, reported by 183 patients (88.8%). It was pleural in nature, exacerbated by coughing, inspiration and change of position in all cases. Initial assessment of chest pain by VAS found a mean intensity of 6±2/10. Dyspnea was reported by 72 patients (35%).

1.2.4. Clinical tolerance of pneumothorax

Poor clinical tolerance of pneumothorax was noted in 32 patients (15.5%). Signs of acute respiratory failure were noted in 31 patients (15%). Hemodynamic damage was noted in only one patient (0.5%).

1.3. Radiological data

1.3.1. Radiological characteristics of pneumothorax

1.3.1.1. Site of pneumothorax

In our series, pneumothorax was right in 120 patients (58.3%), left in 85 patients (41.3%) and bilateral in one patient (0.5%).

1.3.1.2. Pneumothorax size

The following figure (Figure 4) illustrates the distribution of patients by pneumothorax size according to the different learned societies. A statistically significant difference was noted between these three measures (BTS vs ACCP, $p=0.002$; BTS vs SBP, $p<0.001$; ACCP vs SBP, $p<0.001$).

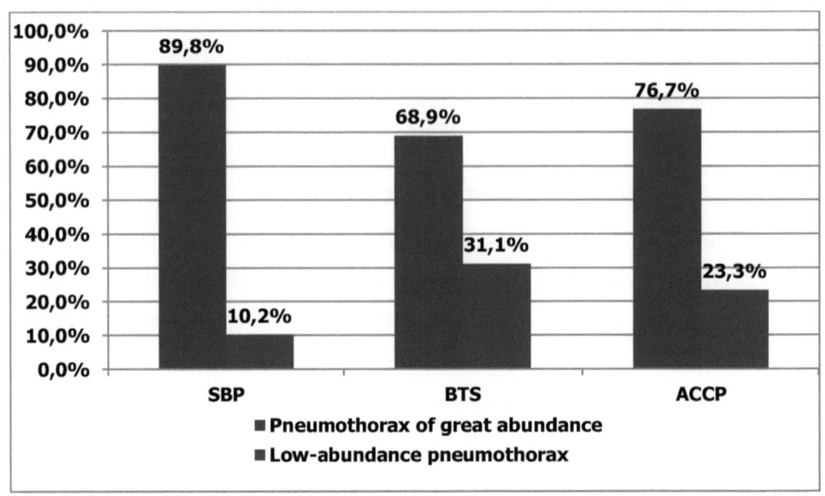

Figure 4: Distribution of patients by pneumothorax size

1.3.1.3. Radiological images in favor of parenchymal pathology

Abnormalities consistent with underlying parenchymal pathology were found in 50 cases (24.3%) (Figure 5).

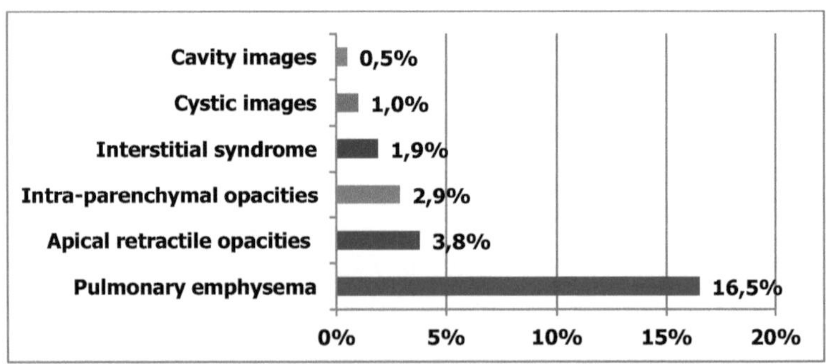

Figure 5: Radiological abnormalities suggestive of underlying parenchymal pathology

1.3.2. Chest CT scan

Chest CT scans were performed in 163 patients (79%) . The mean time to CT scan was 25±76 days [1-702 days] after pneumothorax. It was performed during hospitalization for 75 patients (64.1%) and during follow-up for 28 patients (13.6%).

1.3.2.1. Indications for thoracic CT

Chest CT scans were carried out in 47.8% of cases as part of the etiological assessment of PS (Figure 6).

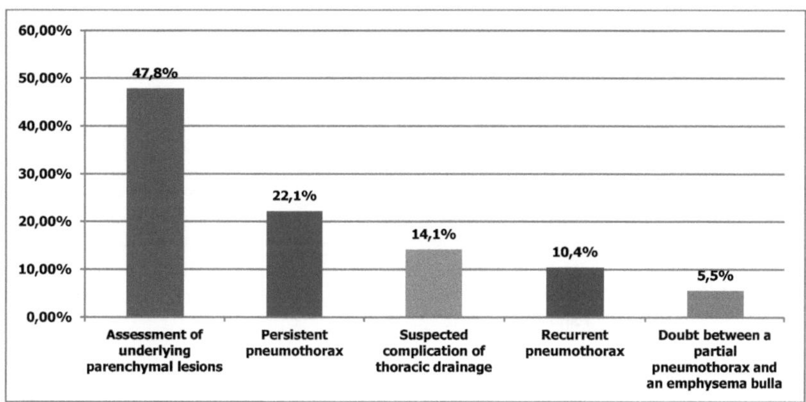

Figure 6: Indications for chest CT in the study population

1.3.2.2. Description of scan anomalies

Parenchymal abnormalities potentially responsible for pneumothorax were noted in 136/163 patients (82.2%) (Figure 7):

- ✓ Blebs in 18/163 patients (11%).
- ✓ Pulmonary emphysema in 114/163 patients (69.9%):
  - ➤ Paraseptal in 101/163 patients (70%)
  - ➤ Centrolobular in 46/163 patients (28.2%)
  - ➤ Panlobular in 19/163 patients (11.7%).
  - ➤ Bullous in 22/163 patients (13.5%)
  - ➤ Several types of emphysema coexisted in 55 patients (33.7%). Emphysema was diffuse and bilateral in 47/114 patients (41.2%), bi-apical in 51/114 patients (44.7%) and unilateral in 16/114 patients (14%).
- ✓ Scarred lobar collapses with bronchial dilatations suggestive of tuberculosis sequelae in 8/163 cases (4.9%).
- ✓ PID with honeycomb images in 4/163 patients (2.5%). SID was already known at the time of pneumothorax in two patients.

- ✓ Single or multiple parenchymal masses in 6/163 patients (3.7%): peripheral tissue mass in 3/163 patients (1.8%), mass with floating membrane in one patient (0.6%) (related to an emesis hydatid cyst) and multiple nodules, some of which are excavated, in 2/163 patients (1.2%).
- ✓ Multiple cystic images in 2/163 patients (1.2%).
- ✓ Cavity image associated with a bronchopleural fistula in one patient (0.6%) with active pulmonary tuberculosis.

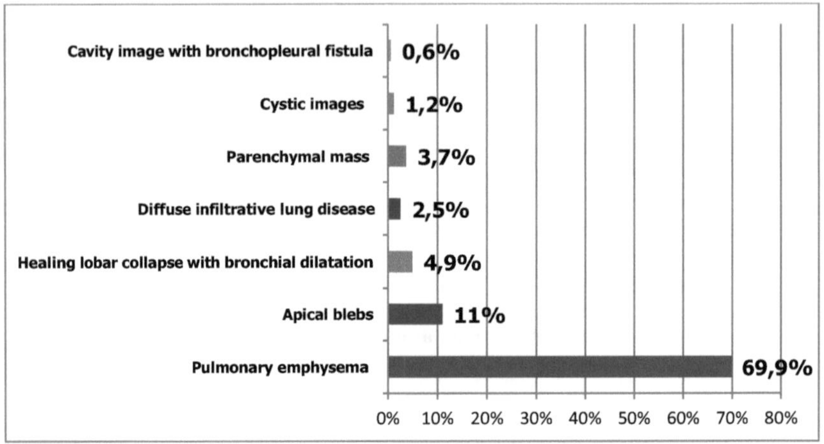

Figure 7: CT abnormalities potentially responsible for pneumothorax

Figures 8 and 9 illustrate the different types of pulmonary emphysema visualized on chest CT.

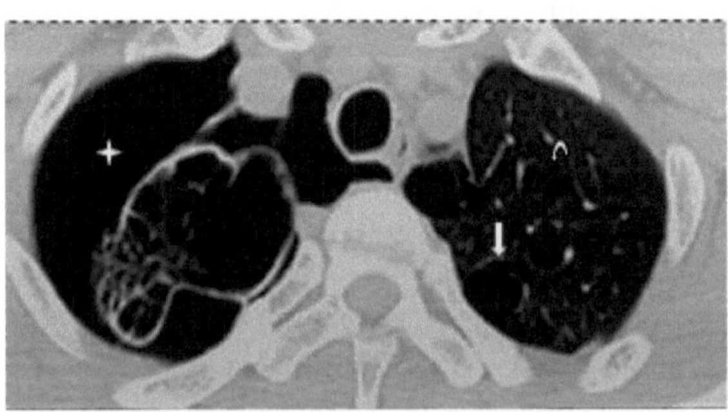

Figure 8: Chest CT scan in parenchymal window and axial section showing right anterior pneumothorax (star) and paraseptal (right arrow) and centrolobular (curved arrow) emphysema.

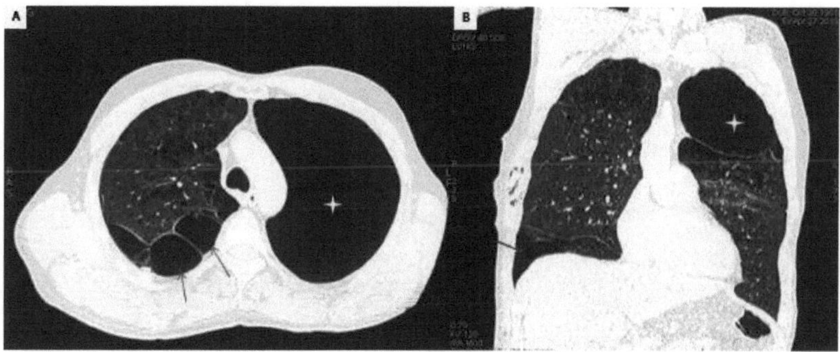

Figure 9: Chest CT scan with parenchymal window and axial (A) and coronal (B) sections showing right pneumothorax (red arrow), bullous (star) and paraseptal emphysema (blue arrow).

Figure 10 shows an example of the sequelae of pulmonary tuberculosis on a chest CT scan.

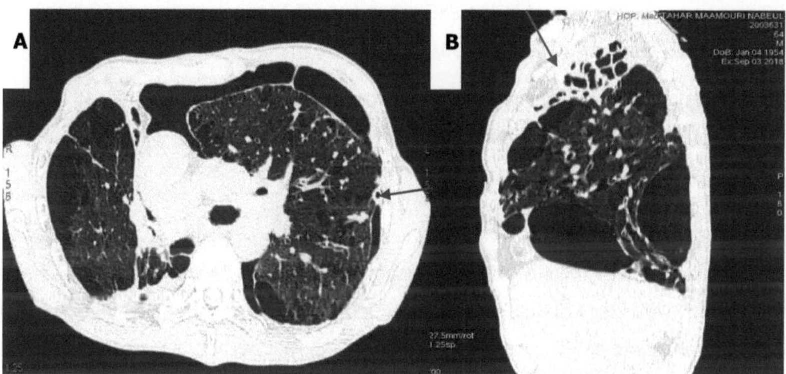

Figure 10: Chest CT scan with parenchymal window and axial (A) and coronal (B) sections showing a left pneumothorax with drain in the pleural cavity (blue arrow), scarring of the right upper lobe with cystic bronchiectasis (red arrow)

1.4. Etiological diagnosis of pneumothorax

Based on clinical and chest X-ray data, the PS was classified (Figure 11):

- ✓ Primitive in 132 patients (64.1%)
- ✓ Secondary in 74 patients (35.9%).

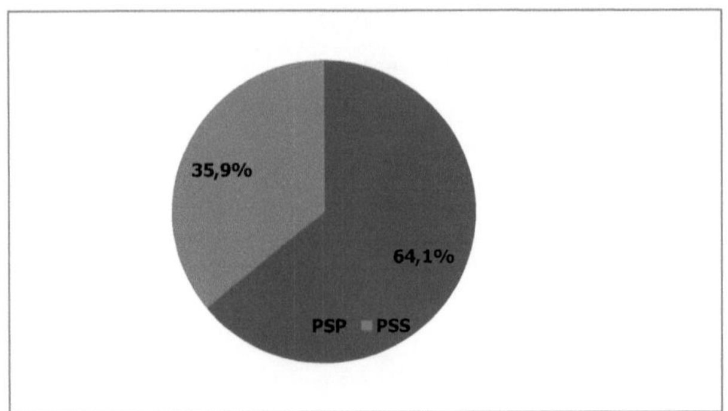

Figure 11: Distribution of primary pneumothoraxes according to etiology

1.4.1. Contribution of CT scans to etiological assessment

Chest CT scans were performed in 93/132 patients in the PSP group (70.4%) (three women and 90 men) and 70/74 patients in the PSS group (94.6%) (one woman and 69 men). It was performed on 4/5 women (80%) and 159/201 (79.1%) men.

Chest CT scans revealed parenchymal abnormalities not visualized on chest X-ray in 65 cases in the PSP group (i.e. 69.9% of patients scanned) and in 44 cases in the PSS group (i.e. 62.8% of patients scanned).

1.4.1.1. In the PSP group

Chest CT scans were normal in 28/93 patients (30.1%) (three women and 23 men). It revealed apical blebs in 16/93 cases (17.2%) (Figure 12). Other parenchymal abnormalities not detected on chest X-ray, such as pulmonary emphysema, were found in 49/93 cases (52.7%). Emphysema was paraseptal in 45 patients, centrolobular in eight and bullous in one. The presence of these anomalies would reclassify the PS as secondary.

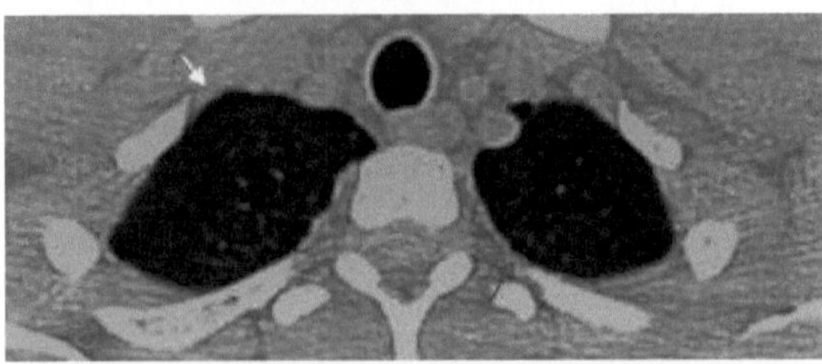

Figure 12: Chest CT scan in axial section and parenchymal window showing a small right anterior pneumothorax (white arrow) and bi-apical blebs (red arrow).

1.4.1.2. In the PSS group

Chest CT scans showed abnormalities consistent with underlying respiratory pathology in all patients. These abnormalities were undetectable on chest X-ray in 31/70 cases (44.3%). Infra-radiological abnormalities included blebs and/or pulmonary emphysema in 31/70 patients (44.3%). Thoracic CT scans therefore enabled a better etiological orientation in these patients.

Figure 13 shows the case of a 45-year-old man with COPD. The frontal chest X-ray showed no significant abnormalities. Axial CT scan shows bullous emphysema in both lungs.

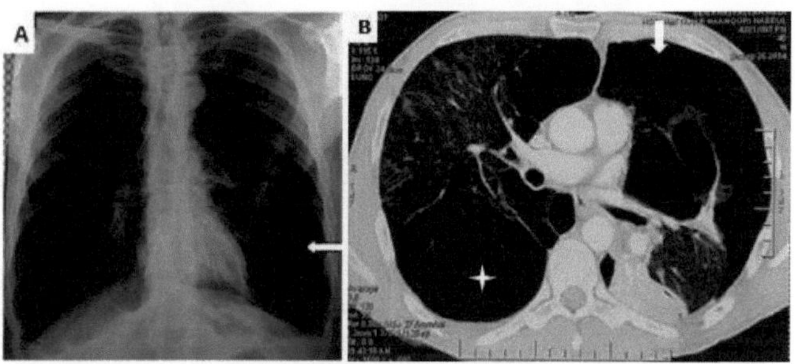

Figure 13: Front thoracic X-ray (A) showing partial left pneumothorax (Arrow). Chest CT scan in axial section and parenchymal window (B) showing left pneumothorax (Arrow) with bullous emphysema in both lungs (Star).

On the other hand, a thoracic CT scan was used to diagnose a vomited hydatid cyst in one patient, demonstrating an excavated parenchymal mass containing a floating membrane . In this case, the chest X-ray showed an opacity of the left pulmonary base.

This examination also enabled a better etiological orientation in two patients with SID, discovered at the time of PS diagnosis, by evoking an emphysema of the apices fibrosis of the bases syndrome in one patient (Figure 14) and a hypersensitivity pneumopathy in a second patient (Figure 15).

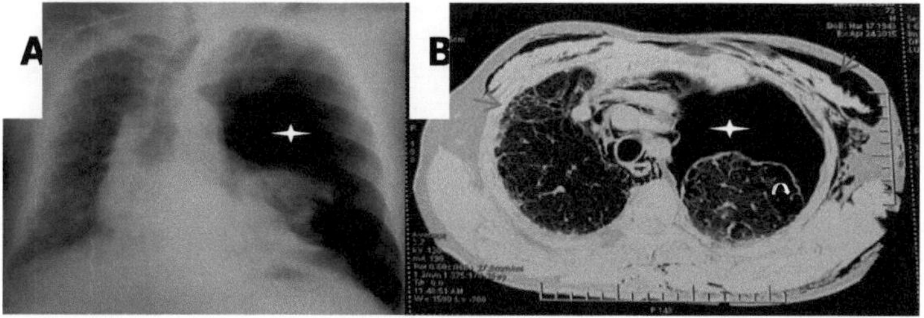

Figure 14: Front thoracic X-ray (A) showing total left pneumothorax with mediastinal deviation towards the contralateral side with interstitial syndrome

on the right lung. Chest CT scan in axial section and parenchymal window (B) showing left pneumothorax (Star), subcutaneous emphysema (Red arrow) associated with paraseptal emphysema (Curved arrow) and honeycomb images (Green arrow)

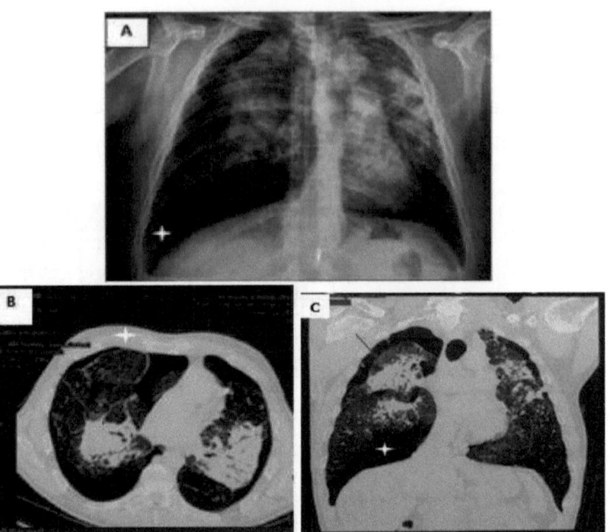

Figure 15: (A)Front chest X-ray showing bilateral opacities of both upper lobes with right pneumothorax (Star) Chest CT scan in axial (B) and coronal (C) sections and parenchymal window showing bilateral pneumothorax in a patient with hypersensitivity pneumopathy

In one patient, primary pulmonary neoplasia was already known at the time of PS diagnosis. For two other patients, this diagnosis was evoked on the thoracic CT scan in the presence of a tissue mass extending into the surrounding structures (Figure 16).

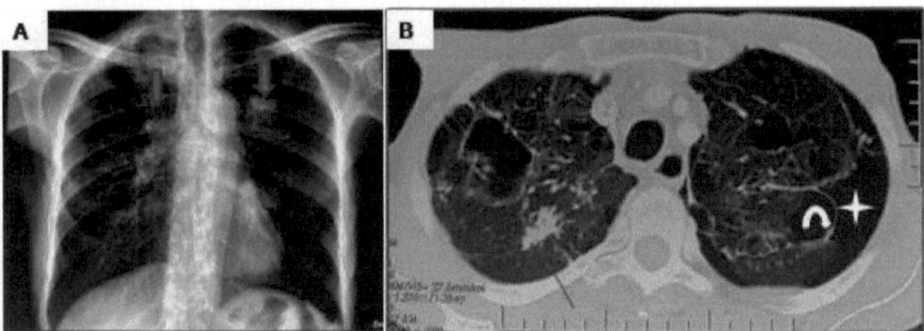

Figure 16: (A) Front-chest X-ray showing left partial pneumothorax (star) associated with intraparenchymal opacities (blue arrow). (B) Chest CT scan in axial sections and parenchymal window showing multiple bilateral parenchymal

tissue processes (blue arrow), bi apical bullous emphysema (curved arrow) and left pneumothorax (star).

In the two patients with extra-thoracic neoplasia, the CT scan suggested that the intra-parenchymal nodules discovered at the time of PS diagnosis were metastatic in nature. Cystic metastases were also observed. The (Figure 17)

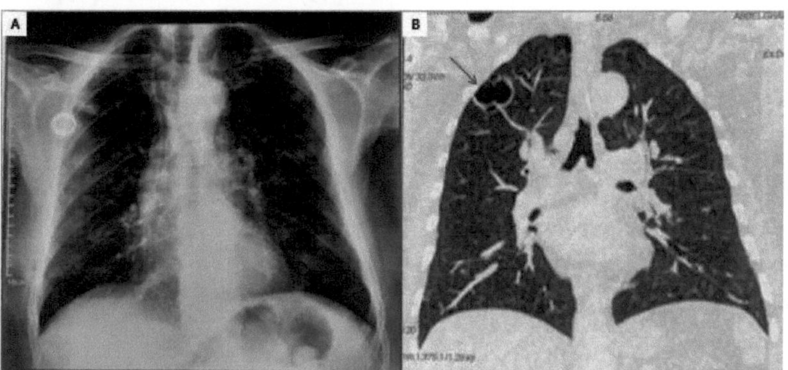

Figure 17: (A) Front thoracic X-ray showing cystic images (red arrow). Chest CT scan in parenchymal window and coronal slices (B) showing cystic metastases (red arrow).

In the case of a patient treated for pulmonary tuberculosis with a cavitary image on the chest X-ray, the CT scan confirmed this diagnosis by showing excavated nodules with a bronchopleural fistula.

Tables I and II summarize the parenchymal radiological abnormalities suggestive of an underlying pulmonary pathology found for patients explored by standard radiography and chest CT in the entire population (Table I) and in the PSS group (Table II).

Table IRadiological and scannographic abnormalities suggestive of underlying pulmonary pathology in patients explored with chest X-ray and chest CT

	Chest X-ray N/Total (%)	Chest CT N/Total (%)
Parenchymal abnormalities	40/163 (24,5)	135/163 (82,8)
Emphysema or blebs	34/163 (20,9)	114/163 (70)
Retractile opacities suggestive of the sequelae of tuberculosis* Scar collapses.**	8/163 (4,9)	8/163 (4,9)
Rounded, excavated opacity Masses or nodules	6/163 (3,7)	6/163 (3,7)
Interstitial syndrome * Diffuse infiltrative pneumonitis ** (DIP)	4/163 (2,5)	4/163 (2,5)
Cavity image	1/163 (0,6)	1/163 (0,6)
Cystic images	2 /163 (1,2)	2/163 (1,2)

*Abnormality detected on chest X-ray** Abnormality detected on chest CT scan

Table III: Radiological abnormalities suggestive of an underlying pulmonary pathology for patients explored by chest CT in the secondary spontaneous pneumothorax group.

	Chest X-ray N/Total (%)	Chest CT N/Total (%)
Parenchymal abnormalities	40/70 (57,1)	70/70 (100)
Emphysema or blebs	34/70 (48,6)	65/70 (92,6)
Retractile opacities suggestive of tuberculosis sequelae*. Healing collapses	8/70 (11,4)	8/70 (11,4)
Opacity Masses or nodules	6/70 (8,6)	6/70 (8,6)
Interstitial syndrome diffuse infiltrative lung disease **, diffuse infiltrative lung disease **, diffuse infiltrative lung disease **, diffuse infiltrative lung disease	4/70 (5,7)	4/70 (5,7)
Cavity image	1/70 (1,4)	1/70 (1,4)
Cystic images	2/70 (2,9)	2 /70 (2,9)

*Anomaly detected on chest X-ray **Anomaly detected on chest CT scan

If scannographic data were taken into account, PS would be classified as primary in 81 cases (39.3%) and secondary in 125 cases (60.6%).

1.4.2. Etiologies of PSS

The etiologies selected for the 74 PSS cases were (Figure 18):

- COPD with pulmonary emphysema in 53 patients, i.e. 25.7% of all PS cases (71.6% of PSS).
- Tuberculosis sequelae in eight patients, i.e. 3.9% of all PS cases (10.8% of PSS).

- Fibrosing PID in four patients (5.4% of PSS):
  - ✓ Idiopathic pulmonary fibrosis: two patients.
  - ✓ Fibrosing hypersensitivity pneumonitis: one patient.
  - ✓ Mediastino-pulmonary sarcoidosis: one patient.
- Active pulmonary tuberculosis in three patients (4.1% of PSS). Pneumothorax occurred after 18 days of anti-tuberculosis treatment in one patient, and was indicative of tuberculosis in two patients.
- Primary bronchopulmonary cancer in three patients (4.1% of PSS).
- Metastatic cystic tumors in two patients (2.7% of PSS).
- Rupture of a pulmonary hydatid cyst in one patient (1.4% of PSS).

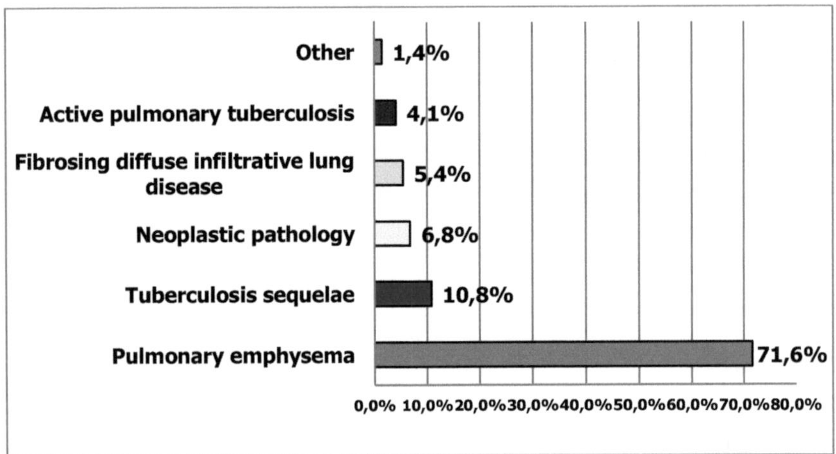

Figure 18: Etiologies of secondary spontaneous pneumothorax

1.5. Therapeutic management

The mean hospital stay was 7.36±4 days [1-30 days].

1.5.1. Conservative treatment

It was recommended for 20 patients with partial pneumothorax and was well tolerated. Return of the lung to the wall was achieved in 18 patients (90%), with a mean delay of 4.75±2 days [2-7 days]. In the remaining two patients, the increased size of the pneumothorax indicated the need for thoracic drainage.

1.5.2. Pleural evacuation

1.5.2.1. Needle exsufflation

Exsufflation was recommended in three patients. The lung returned to the wall in two patients. Chest drainage was necessary in 3ème patients when exsufflation failed.

1.5.2.2. Chest drainage

Thoracic drainage was performed in 185 patients (90%):

- 178/185 (96.2%) patients with total PS: 114 patients in the PSP group and 64 patients in the PSS group.
- 7/185 patients with partial PS before :
    - ✓ Failed exsufflation in a patient with PSP.
    - ✓ Radiological worsening after conservative treatment in two patients with PSS related to emphysematous lung.
    - ✓ Poorly tolerated pneumothorax in two patients with PSS (sequelae of tuberculosis: one patient; bullous emphysema: one patient).
    - ✓ Recurrent pneumothorax secondary to primary pulmonary neoplasia in two patients.

The mean duration of thoracic drainage was 6.3±3 days [8- 22 days].

1.5.3. Medical pleurodesis

- Medical pleurodesis through the drain was performed for 13/206 patients (6.3%) with PSS (A persistent pneumothorax 7 patients and recurrent for 6 other patients).
- Surgical pleurodesis was indicated in 35/206 patients (17%) (persistent pneumothorax in 19 patients, recurrent pneumothorax in 13 patients, bilateral pneumothorax in one patient and hemopneumothorax in two patients).
- Preoperative chest CT showed parenchymal abnormalities in 29/35 cases (82.9%), with blebs in 3/35 patients (8.6%), pulmonary emphysema in 25/35 patients (71.4%), PID in 2/35 patients (5.7%) and ruptured hydatid cysts in 1/35 patients (2.9%).
- The surgical procedures associated with pleurodesis were :
    - ✓ Bullae resection in 16/35 patients (45.7%): 4/16 patients (25%) in the PSP group and 12/19 patients (63.2%) in the PSS group.

- ✓ Bleb resection in 1/35 patients (2.9%) in the PSP group.
- ✓ A cure for a pulmonary hydatid cyst for one patient (2.9%).
- ✓ Surgical lung biopsy for patients with CT scans suggestive of PHS (2.9%).

- The preoperative CT scan showed emphysema lesions and/or blebs in 15 patients (88.2%) of those who underwent bubble or bleb resection (n=17). It oriented the biopsy site for the patient with a PHS and guided the operative procedure for the patient with a ruptured hydatid cyst.

1.6. Long-term trends

- The mean duration of follow-up of patients after hospital discharge was 2±1 years [1y-3y]. During follow-up, PS recurrence was observed in 16 patients (7.76%) within 171±242 days [7-803 days]. Recurrence was homolateral in 12 cases (75%) and contralateral in four (25%).
- Smoking cessation was successful in 75 patients (36.4%). Persistent exposure to passive smoking was noted in 39 patients (18.9%).
- No chronic respiratory signs were noted during the follow-up period in patients in the PSP group with scannographic abnormalities of pulmonary emphysema unrecognized on chest X-ray.

2. Analytical study

2.1. Socio-demographic characteristics

2.1.1. Age

- The mean age of patients was older in the PSS group than in the PSP group (60.6 ± 12 years [22-87 years] versus 29 ± 9 years [16-50 years]; $p<0.001$).
- In the PSP group, the mean age was older in men than in women (30 ± 9 years versus 22.7 ± 4 years), with no statically significant difference (p=0.1). Ninety-four percent of patients (n=124) with PSP were under 45 years of age.
- In the PSS group, the mean age was older in men than in women (61 versus 22 years; p=0.001).

2.1.2. Type

Men accounted for 96.9% of PSP cases (128 cases) and 98.6% of PSS cases (73 cases) (p=0.65).

2.1.3. Smoking

- The frequency of active smoking was comparable between the PSP and PSS groups (114 patients (86.4%) versus 69 patients (93.2%); p=0.13)
- Average smoking habits were higher in the PSS group than in the PSP group (42 ± 21 PA versus 16 ± 14 PA; p<0.001).

2.1.4. Anthropometric data

- Mean BMI was lower in the PSP group than in the PSS group (20.4±2 kg/m2 versus 22.4±4 kg/m2 ; p=0.002).
- On average, patients in the PSP group were taller than those in the PSS group (1.757 ± 0.072 meters [1.57- 1.93] versus 1.7 ± 0.066 meters [1.59- 1.94]; p<0.001).
- The longline morphotype was more frequently found in the PSP group than in the PSS group (36 patients or 27.3% versus nine patients or 12.2%; p=0.012).

2.2. Clinical data

- The average consultation time was shorter in the PSP group than in the PSS group (33 ± 44 hours versus 64 ± 81 hours; p=0.001).
- Chest pain was more frequent in the PSP group than in the PSS group (127 patients (96.2%) versus 56 patients (75.6%); p<0.001). Dyspnea was more frequently reported by patients in the PSS group than by patients in the PSP group (34 patients (45.9%) versus 38 patients (28.7%); p=0.013).
- Respiratory impairment was more frequently noted in the PSS group than in the PSP group (27 patients (36.5%) versus four patients (3%); p<0.001). Hemodynamic damage was noted in only one patient in the PSS group.

2.3. Radiological data

Chest CT scans were performed in 93 patients in the PSP group (70.5%) and in 70 patients in the PSS group (94.6%) (p<0.001). It was performed 26 ± 60 days [1-360 days] after the occurrence of pneumothorax in the PSP group and 25 ± 94 days [1-702 days] after the diagnosis of pneumothorax in the PSS group. This scan was performed :

- During hospitalization for 80.6% of patients in the PSP group (n=75) and for 87.1% of patients in the PSS group (n=61).
- At the follow-up visit for 18 patients in the PSP group and nine patients in the PSS group (p=0.26).

2.3.1. Thoracic CT scan indications according to PS etiology (Figure 19)

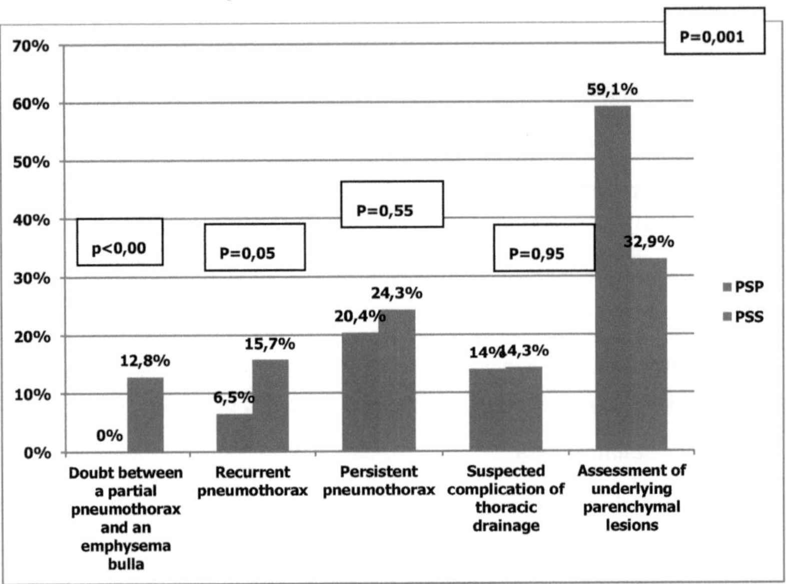

Figure 19: Distribution of spontaneous pneumothorax according to indications for thoracic CT scan

2.3.2. Description of scan anomalies

- Parenchymal abnormalities potentially causing pneumothorax were noted in 65/93 patients (69.9%) in the PSP group and in 70/70 patients in the PSS group (100%) (p=0.001) .
- Blebs were more frequent in the PSP group (16/93 patients (17.2%) in the PSP group versus 2/70 patients (2.9%) in the PSS group; p<0.001).
- Pulmonary emphysema was more frequently found in the PSS group (65/70 patients (92.9%) versus 49/93 patients (52.7%); p<0.001) (Figure 20).

- Emphysema was diffuse and bilateral in 7/49 patients (14.3%) in the PSP group and 40/65 patients (61.5%) in the PSS group (p<0.001), bi-apical in 32/49 patients (65.3%) in the PSP group and 19/65 patients in the PSS group (p<0.001) and unilateral in 10/49 patients (20.4%) in the PSP group and 5/65 patients (7.8%) in the PSS group (p=0.05).

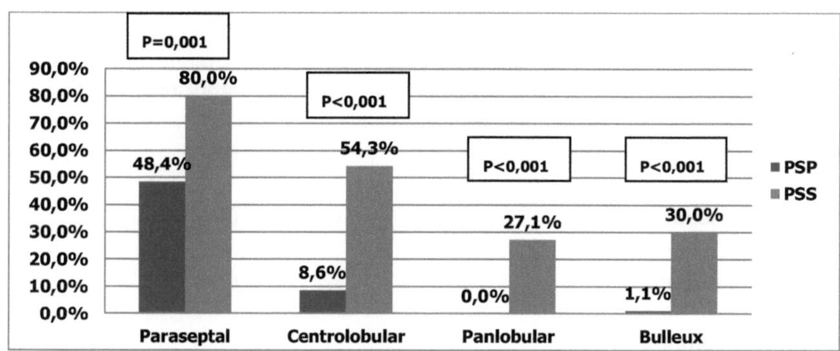

Figure 20: Distribution of spontaneous pneumothoraxes according to the type of emphysema described on chest CT.

1.1. Therapeutic data (Figure 21)

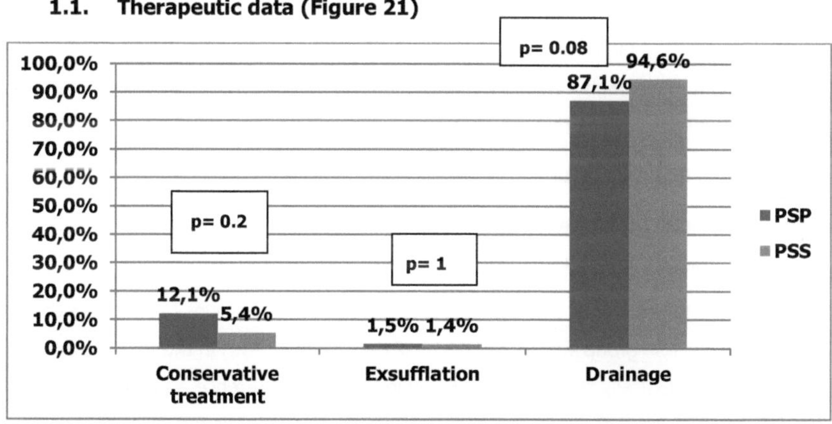

Figure 21: Distribution of spontaneous pneumothoraxes according to treatment modality

The mean duration of chest drainage was shorter in the PSP group than in the PSS group (5.7 ± 3 days versus 7.3 ± 3 days; p=0.001). Average hospital stay was shorter in the PSP group than in the PSS group (6.6 ± 3 days versus 8.7 ± 5.3 days; p=0.002).

Medical pleurodesis through the drain was performed in 13 patients in the PSS group. Surgical pleurodesis was recommended in 19 patients in the PSP group (14.4%) and in 16 patients in the PSS group (21.6%) (p=0.3). Table IV illustrates the indications for pleurodesis according to whether the pneumothorax was primary or secondary.

Table IIIIndications for pleurodesis depending on whether spontaneous pneumothorax is primary or secondary

Indication for surgical pleurodesis	Primary spontaneous pneumothorax N (%)	Secondary spontaneous pneumothorax N (%)	p
Persistent pneumothorax	9 (47,4)	14 (48,3)	0,9
Recurrent pneumothorax	9 (47,4)	13 (44,8)	0,8
Hemopneumothorax	1 (5,3)	1 (3,4)	1
Bilateral pneumothorax	0	1 (3,4)	1

All patients underwent preoperative chest CT. Parenchymal abnormalities discovered on this scan were more frequent in the PSS group (16/16 patients (100%) versus 13/19 patients (68.4%); p=0.02). Blebs were found only in patients in the PSP group (3/19 patients (15.8%)). Pulmonary emphysema was found to be comparable in both groups (10/19 patients (76.9%) in the PSP group versus 15/16 patients in the PSS group (93.8 %); p=0.29).

1.2. Scalable data

- PS recurrences were more frequent in the PSS group (11 patients (14.9%) versus five patients (3.8%); p=0.004).

The mean time to recurrence was comparable between the two groups (117.8 ± 85 days [24-220 days] in the PSP group versus 199.8 ± 287 days [7-803 days] in the PSS group; p=0.5). There was no statistically significant relationship between recurrence and patient age (0% if age<20 years, 31.2% if age between 20 and 40 years, 43.8% if age between 40 and 60 years and 25% if age >60 years; (p=0.13). Recurrence of PS was not correlated either with smoking intoxication (13.6% in non-smokers versus 7.1% in smokers; p=0.39) or with continued smoking (8% in case of continued smoking versus 16.7% in case of cessation; p=0.2). There was no correlation between pneumothorax recurrence and lanky morphotype (13.6% if weight/height ≥ 3 cm/Kg versus 6.2% if weight/height ≤ 3cm/Kg; p=0.11). Mean BMI was not correlated with the risk of recurrence (19.6 kg/m^2 in case of recurrence versus 21.17 kg/m^2 in absence of recurrence; p=0.19). No statistically significant relationship was noted between PS recurrence and the presence of blebs on chest CT, nor with the presence of emphysematous lesions, their location and type. Table V summarizes the various factors correlated with the risk of recurrence of spontaneous pneumothorax.

Table IVFactors correlated with the risk of recurrence of spontaneous pneumothorax

		Recurrence of spontaneous pneumothorax		p
		No N (%)	Yes N (%)	
Presence of blebs		18 (22,8)	0 (0)	0,3
Presence of emphysema		102 (68,9)	12 (80)	0,5
Location of emphysema lesions	**Bi-apical**	32 (30,2)	3 (27,3)	1
	Two upper lobes	16 (15,1)	0 (0)	0,35
	Diffuse bilateral	4 (37,7)	7 (63,6)	0,1
	Unilateral	15 (14,2)	1 (9,1)	1
Type of emphysema	**Paraseptal**	91 (61,5)	10 (66,7)	0,6
	Centrolobular	41 (27,9)	5 (33,3)	0,7
	Panlobular	16 (10,8)	3 (20)	0,3
	Bulleux	18 (12,2)	4 (26,7)	0,1

1.3. Summary and comparison between PSP and PSS

Table VI provides a comparative summary of clinical and therapeutic data for the PSP and PSS groups.

Table V Comparative table of clinical and therapeutic data for the primary and secondary spontaneous pneumothorax groups.

	Primary spontaneous pneumothorax	Secondary spontaneous pneumothorax	P
Age (years)	29 ± 9	60,6 ± 12	**<0,001**
Active smoker (%)	86,4	93,2	0,13
Male gender (%)	96,9	98,6	0,65
Longline morphotype (%)	27,3	12,2	**0,012**
Consultation time (hours)	33	64	**0,001**
Chest pain (%)	96,2	75,6	**<0,001**
Dyspnea (%)	28,7	45,9	**0,013**
Acute respiratory failure (%)	3	36,5	**<0,001**
Chest drainage (%)	87,1	94,6	0,08
Drainage time (days)	5 ± 3	8 ± 4	0,1
Drainage complications	47/115 (40,9%)	45/70 (64,3%)	**0,002**
Recurrence (%)	3,8	14,9	**0,004**

D ISCUSSION

PS is a frequent occurrence in pneumology. Classically, PSP occurs in young subjects with apparently healthy lungs on the basis of clinical findings and chest X-ray, whereas PSS occurs in pathological lungs. Distinguishing between these two entities is essential, as it guides management. It has now been established that the thoracic CT scan is the most effective radiological examination for studying the lung parenchyma. It provides a precise lesion assessment, highlighting abnormalities that may be overlooked on the chest X-ray, and thus enables a better etiological classification of pneumothorax [10]. However, the role of CT in the etiological investigation of this condition remains controversial. In this context, we conducted a prospective study of 206 patients hospitalized for PS at the Pneumology Department of Mohamed Taher Mâamouri Hospital in Nabeul between August 2013 and December 2019 with the aim of determining the etiological profile of PS and identifying the place of chest CT in the etiological investigation of this condition as well as in its therapeutic management.

In our study, PSS was defined according to the BTS recommendations published in 2010, as a PS occurring in subjects aged over 50 with a history of heavy smoking or with clinical signs or chest radiography abnormalities in favor of an underlying respiratory pathology. [1].

The mean age of our population was 40 ± 18 years [16-87]. Pathologies predisposing to PS were noted in 51 patients (24.7%): COPD in 36 patients (17.5%), active pulmonary tuberculosis in three patients (1.4%) and cured with parenchymal sequelae in nine patients (4.3%), fibrosing IPD in two patients (1%) and primary bronchopulmonary cancer in one patient. Chest X-rays, taken for all patients on admission, showed parenchymal abnormalities consistent with underlying pulmonary pathology in 50 cases (24.2%). These abnormalities were represented by pulmonary emphysema in 34 patients (16.5%), apical retractile opacity with areolar images suggestive of tuberculosis sequelae in eight cases (3.8%), intra-parenchymal round opacities in six patients (2.9%), cystic images in two patients (1%) and cavitary images in one patient (0.5%), and interstitial syndrome in four patients (1.9%). In our study, we identified 132 cases of PSP (64.1%) and 74 cases of PSS (35.9%), based on clinical and chest X-ray data. Chest CT scans were performed in 163 patients (79.1%) (93 in the PSP group and 70 in the PSS group). It was indicated as part of the etiological work-up for PS in 78 patients (47.8%). In the PSP group, the thoracic CT scan revealed infra-radiological lesions potentially incriminating in the occurrence of PS in 65 cases (70%), such as apical blebs in 16/93 cases (17.2%) and pulmonary emphysema in 49/93 patients (52.7%). In the PSS group, the abnormalities likely to have caused PS were pulmonary emphysema in

65/70 patients (92.8%), and pulmonary tuberculosis sequelae such as cicatricial lobar collapse and bronchial dilatation in 8/70 patients (11.4%), PID with honeycomb images in 4/70 patients (5.7%), cystic metastases in two patients (2.9%), an emesis hydatid cyst in one patient (1.4%), an excavated tumor mass in three patients (4.3%) and a cavitary image associated with a bronchopleural fistula in one patient (1.4%). Emphysema lesions were infra-radiological in 31 patients (44.3%). In our series, COPD with pulmonary emphysema topped the list of etiologies for PSS (53 cases, 71.6%), followed by sequelae of pulmonary tuberculosis (eight cases, 10.8%). Pleurodesis was performed in 48 patients (23.3%). Pleurodesis was performed medically in 13 patients (6.3% of cases), and surgically in the remaining 35 (17%). All surgical patients (n=35 ;17%) (19 in the PSP group and 16 in the PSS group) underwent a chest CT scan as part of their preoperative work-up. This examination showed more frequent parenchymal abnormalities in patients in the PSS group (100% versus 68.4%; p=0.02), such as blebs in 3/19 patients in the PSP group (15.8%), pulmonary emphysema in 25 patients (10/19 patients in the PSP group (76.9%) and 15/16 patients in the PSS group (93.8%); p=0.29), PID in 2/16 patients in the PSS group (12.5%) and pulmonary hydatidosis in one patient in the PSS group (6.3%). The surgical procedures associated with pleurodesis were bullae resection in 16/35 patients (45.7%), bleb resection in 1/35 patients (2.9%), cure of a pulmonary hydatid cyst in one patient (2.9%) and surgical lung biopsy in the patient with a CT scan suggestive of PHS (2.9%). The preoperative CT scan had described emphysematous bullae in 15 patients (88.2%) of those who underwent resection of bullae or blebs (n=17) and directed the site of biopsy for the patient with PHS. The average follow-up time of patients after hospital discharge was 2 ± 1 years [1 year - 3 years]. None of the patients in the PSP group with parenchymal abnormalities on chest CT such as pulmonary emphysema presented clinical signs in favor of respiratory pathology during the follow-up period. Pneumothorax recurrence was observed in 16 patients (7.76%) more often in the PSS group than in the PSP group (14.9% versus 3.8%; p=0.004). No correlation was observed between patient age, morphotype, presence of blebs or emphysematous lesions, their location and type on chest CT, and recurrence of PS.

Highlights of our study

- Its forward-looking nature
- A study period extended by six and a half years.
- A relatively large sample size

To our knowledge, this is the first nationwide study to compare the contribution of CT scans with that of chest X-rays in distinguishing between the primary and secondary origins of PS.

Weaknesses of our study

- Its monocentric nature.
- Chest CT scans were performed according to specific indications and not routinely for all patients.
- The analysis of scan data, in particular of pulmonary emphysema, was performed qualitatively without using a scoring system to assess the extent of lesions.

Etiological diagnosis of spontaneous pneumothorax

PS is a common pathology in pneumology. It has been responsible for 9.1 to 14.1 hospitalizations per 100,000 per year over the past fifty years. In a study carried out in France, involving all patients hospitalized for PS between 2008 and 2011, the annual incidence of this condition was 22.7 per 100,000 inhabitants. In Europe, the annual incidence of PSP was estimated at 18-24 cases per 100,000 inhabitants [6[6-9] and that of PSP and PSS combined was 16.8 per 100,000 inhabitants in England (24 per 100,000 inhabitants for men and 9.8 per 100,000 inhabitants for women) [14, 15]. In our study, the annual incidence of SP was 29 cases/year.

Distinguishing between PSP and PSS is essential, as it guides therapeutic management. In practice, the distinction between the two types of PSP is based on the clinical picture and the chest radiograph. [1]. Epidemiologically, certain characteristics differentiate PSP from PSS. PSP is the most common type of SP, accounting for 80% of cases in the study by Ferraro et al. [16] and 70% of cases in the study by Brown et al. [20]. It is three times more frequent than PSS [18]. As in our study, several other authors have confirmed the high prevalence of PSP compared with PSS. Table VII summarizes the frequency of spontaneous pneumothorax according to whether it is primary or secondary in various studies.

Table VI Frequency of spontaneous pneumothorax according to its primary and secondary nature in various studies

	PSP	PSS
Bobbio [12]	85%	15%
Onuki [19]	65,1%	34,9%
Brown [20]	69,7%	30,3%
Tanaka [21]	34%	66%
Weissberg [17]	30,2%	69,8%
Ruppert [22]	41%	59%
Hallifax [23]	39,2%	60,8%
Our study	64,1%	35,9%

PSP typically affects younger patients, with a mean age varying, in the literature, between 27 and 35 years, whereas PSS classically affects subjects over 50 years of age. Bobbio et al, in a series of 42595 patients hospitalized for PS, found a higher mean age for PSS than PSP (53 ± 20 versus 35 ± 18; $p<0.0001$) [1, 12]. This bimodal distribution was demonstrated by a large study including all patients aged over 15 hospitalized for PS between 1968 and 2016 in England, with a first frequency peak between 15 and 34 for PSP and a second peak over 60 for PSS. In fact, lung pathologies are more frequent in adults over 50, and smoking, quantified as PA, is more important with advancing age. According to the literature, the peak frequency of PSP is later in women than in men (40 years for women versus 20 years for men) [6, 7, 12]. This could be explained by the earlier and more frequent onset of smoking in men compared with women [15, 22]. In line with the literature, the mean age of our population was lower for the PSP group than for the PSS group (29 ± 9 years versus 60.6 ± 12 years; $p<0.001$). However, the mean age for the PSP group was greater for men than for women (29.8 ± 9 years versus 22.7 ± 4 years; $p=0.1$). The greater number of men than women in our study population could represent a statistical bias. Primary or secondary SP mainly affects males. This clear male predominance has been demonstrated by numerous authors, with a male/female gender ratio ranging from 2.9 to 6.27 [7, 10, 12, 14, 15]. Our results were consistent with the literature, with 97% of PSP and 99% of PSS occurring in men. This could be explained by the high prevalence and early onset of smoking in men compared with women. In Tunisia, smoking affects 55.4% of men and only 4% of women [26].

Currently, smoking is the main environmental risk factor contributing to the onset and recurrence of PSP, increasing the risk of its occurrence by a factor of 22 for men and nine for women. This risk is correlated with the duration of tobacco intoxication and daily PA consumption. In fact, smoking is incriminated in the genesis of respiratory bronchiolitis, favoring the formation of bubbles and the occurrence of pneumothorax. In the case of PSS, smoking is also implicated in the development of underlying respiratory pathology [18,19,25]. Our results confirm the close link between smoking and the onset of PSS: 89% of our patients were smokers (86.4% of patients in the PSP group and 93.2% in the PSS group; p=0.13), with an average daily consumption of 27 ± 22 PA. Cannabis consumption was also incriminated in the occurrence of PS. Cannabis inhalation accelerates lung parenchymal destruction. Its effect seems to intensify that of tobacco [27]. In our study, only nine of our patients (4.3%) were cannabis smokers, but our data may suffer from an underestimation bias, since it is common not to declare the use of this drug for fear of prejudice and because it is illegal in our country.

PSP classically affects smokers of large stature with a low BMI [12]. Pathophysiologically, pleural pressure is more negative at the lung apices than at the bases. In tall people, this distension force predisposes to the development of blebs on the lung surface. When these blebs rupture as a result of increased pressure within the lung, the result is pneumothorax. Air leaks from the ruptured bubble into the pleural cavity [26, 33, 34]. Other hypotheses have been put forward in the literature to explain the occurrence of PSP. Some authors have suggested the possibility of diffuse inflammatory disease of the visceral pleura, with an increase in its porosity [18]. This inflammation would lead to destabilization of the mesothelial cells in the visceral pleura, which would be replaced by an inflammatory elastofibrotic layer with increased porosity, allowing air to leak from the lung into the pleural space [26, 35]. Another possibility is an imbalance in the protease-antiprotease balance, with overexpression of matrix metalloproteinases 2, 7 and 9 in patients with PSP. This was demonstrated by immunohistochemistry on pleural samples from 50 patients operated on for PSP versus a control group including patients with bronchopulmonary cancer [32]. PSS can be explained by two mechanisms: rupture due to tension in sub-pleural air structures that have exceeded their own compliance (blebs, bubbles, air cysts), or the extension of a parenchymal necrosis process to the pleura, leading to erosion and subsequent rupture of the latter, and the creation of a broncho-pleural fistula, particularly during necrotizing or cystic processes of the pulmonary parenchyma. [18].

Classically, pneumothorax is revealed by one or more of the following signs: pleural stitch or stab-type chest pain, exacerbated by coughing or changing position, dyspnea and irritative dry cough [29, 30]. Chest pain is the most frequent symptom in PSP, reported in an average of 69.2% of cases in the literature, followed by dyspnoea, present in an average of 54.5% of cases [11]. In the case of PSS, dyspnea is the main symptom. In a series of 112 men with PSP, Voge et al found the notion of chest pain in 89% of cases, while dyspnea was present in only 61%. [34]. In the series by Abolnik et al, who studied cases of PSP, chest pain was also the most frequent symptom, found in 95% of cases, followed by dyspnoea in 77.1%. [35]. In the study by Tanaka et al, dyspnoea was present in 64.2% of PSS cases, whereas it was present in only 10.2% of PSP cases ($p < 0.01$) [21]. In PSP, functional symptoms are usually moderate or sometimes completely absent. They usually subside within a few days of the pneumothorax. [9]. In our study, pain was the most frequent symptom, found in 90% of cases more frequently in PSP than in PSS (96.2% versus 75.6%; $p<0.001$), followed by dyspnea in 35% of cases. Similar to the literature, dyspnea was more frequent in PSS than in PSP (45.9% versus 28.7%; $p= 0.013$).

PSP is usually better tolerated than PSS. Hypoxemia alone or associated with hypercapnia, as well as acute respiratory failure or hemodynamic impairment, which are rare in PSP, are often found in PSS because of low cardiopulmonary reserve due to the underlying respiratory pathology. [8, 26]. Tanaka et al found a lower mean PaO_2 in patients with PSS compared with those with PSP (PSS: 62.1mmHg and PSP: 81.2 mm Hg) [21]. Brown et al noted desaturation <92% room air on arrival in 2% of PSP cases and 20% of PSS cases ($p<0.0001$) [20]. Our results were in line with the literature, and acute respiratory failure was more frequently found in cases of PSS (36.5% versus 3%; $p<0.001$).

The role of chest CT in the etiological diagnosis of spontaneous pneumothorax

Thanks to its high spatial and contrast resolution, chest CT offers a finer semiological analysis of the lung parenchyma than chest X-ray. It allows better characterization of underlying parenchymal lesions in cases of PS, and sometimes detects abnormalities that may go unnoticed on chest radiography [36,37]. Indeed, many authors have confirmed the existence of underlying parenchymal lesions in PSP, such as emphysematous lesions. For example, Lesur et al. demonstrated the presence of peripheral subpleural emphysema in 80% of cases and centrilobular emphysema in 60% of cases, using chest CT scans of 20 patients with PSP judged to be primary on the basis of clinical examination and chest X-ray findings. The author concludes that CT scanning is more sensitive than standard chest radiography in detecting emphysematous lesions, and that only prolonged follow-up of these patients will determine whether these lesions are the cause of chronic respiratory disease. [29]. This was also demonstrated by the prospective study by Ruppert et al, who found emphysematous lesions in 51.8% of chest scans performed on 83 patients with PSP. These lesions were more frequent in cannabis and tobacco smokers than in tobacco-only smokers (71.9% and 50% of cases respectively). The authors conclude that chest CT scans in patients with PSP who smoke tobacco and/or cannabis could be useful for early detection of emphysema lesions and to encourage these patients to quit smoking. [25].

In 1993, Bense et al. demonstrated the presence of localized areas of lower density lung parenchyma, delimited by a very thin wall, called "emphysematous-type changes" in 81% of PSP cases, whereas such images were present in only 20% of the control group. The latter group included apparently healthy subjects who had never smoked [38]. Bintcliffe et al compared the scans of a first group of PSP patients with a second group of control patients. They found that the extent of emphysema and the percentage of low-density parenchymal areas were greater in the PSP group compared with the control group, with a statically significant difference (median 0.25% versus 0%; p= 0.019 [39].

Cross-sectional imaging is also more sensitive than chest radiography for identifying blebs, which are visible on scannographic sections as soon as their diameter reaches 3 mm, whereas they are only visible on chest radiography from a diameter of 10 mm onwards [38]. Blebs and subpleural bullae were detected in 50-80% of chest scans performed on patients with PSP [18,39]. Mitlehner also demonstrated, in his prospective study of 35 patients with PSP, the superiority of chest CT over chest X-ray in the detection of subpleural blebs. These abnormalities were detected in 31 cases on chest CT, whereas they were highlighted on only 11 chest X-rays [41]. In the study by Kobayashi et al, sub pleural blebs and apical linear opacities were significantly more frequent on CT scans in the PSP group than in the control group. [42]. Histologically, these apical opacities corresponded to fibrosis, pleural thickening and band atelectasis associated with foci of alveolar collapse. The sensitivity of thoracic CT to detect these abnormalities is better when the scanner used is high-resolution with thin sections, and reviews both axial and coronal sections [43, 44]. Thoracic CT can also show abnormalities in the configuration of the thorax, which is more common in patients with PSP.

According to the retrospective study by C.H Park et al, patients with PSP had a thorax that was flatter anteroposteriorly, narrower laterally and longer craniocaudally, compared with a control group including age- and sex-matched healthy subjects [45]. These biogeometric features are thought to be associated with the formation of subpleural bubbles, the rupture of which is at the origin of PSP.

Thoracic CT is also the best examination for studying diffuse infiltrative pathologies. It can detect infra-radiological interstitial lesions in symptomatic patients with confirmed PID in 10-15% of cases [46]. In our study, in two cases, PS was a complication of an already known IDP, and in two others, it was indicative of this pathology. In both cases, the chest X-ray was abnormal, necessitating a thoracic CT scan. This examination enabled a better etiological orientation of the PS, showing an appearance compatible with PHS in one case and with a syndrome of emphysema of the apices and fibrosis of the bases in the other case.

It is also the technique of choice for detecting cystic pathologies of the lung parenchyma. These lesions are often complicated by PS and may go undetected on chest radiography [47,48]. In a Chinese population, Birt-Hogg-Dubbé syndrome was discovered in 10% of patients with PSP on chest CT. This led to early diagnosis of the renal tumors often associated with this syndrome, enabling better treatment of this rare entity and consequently a better prognosis [49]. Lymphangioleiomyomatosis is a rare pathology that causes PS in women. It is often only discovered in recurrent cases. Some authors suggest a systematic thoracic CT scan for PSP in women aged between 25 and 54 years, in order to avoid overlooking this rare entity and to be able to propose pleurodesis, which is recommended as soon as the first episode of PS occurs, due to the high risk of recurrence. [50,51]. In our series, cystic lesions were identified on the chest X-ray of two patients with PSS. Chest CT scans suggested the malignant nature of these abnormalities.

Based on the above findings, many authors have proposed a systematic thoracic CT scan in the face of a first episode of PS in order to adapt its management, which differs according to the learned societies depending on its primary or secondary nature [22]. Thus, in its recommendations published in 2010, the BTS envisages outpatient management with simple monitoring only in the case of a small (<2cm), asymptomatic PS with no evidence of chronic respiratory pathology. Similarly, needle exsufflation is possible for PSP larger than 2 cm and/or symptomatic, whereas thoracic drainage must be performed for PSS with these same characteristics [1,22]. According to the ACCP, hospitalization is recommended for a small PSS, even without clinical repercussions, whereas outpatient management can be envisaged for a PSS with the same characteristics. [7]. Nevertheless, the literature is not unanimous on the value of routine chest CT scans for every first episode of SP. Indeed, lesions discovered by CT scan, particularly emphysematous lesions found in patients with PSP, are not necessarily synonymous with underlying respiratory disease. Added to this is the fact that this examination is not always easily accessible, and exposes the patient to excess cost and irradiation compared with chest radiography [9,52]. To date, the systematic performance of a chest CT scan in the face of a first episode of PS has not been recommended by the learned societies. It is only indicated, as part of its etiological investigation, in cases of doubt about an underlying pulmonary pathology, without guidance from clinical and chest X-ray data [1,7]. In our study, pulmonary emphysema lesions were found in 52.7% of PSP cases investigated by chest CT. In such cases, it would be legitimate to ask whether these abnormalities would be predisposing lesions for chronic obstructive respiratory diseases such as COPD. However, none of these patients developed signs suggestive of such a pathology during the study period.

There are many etiologies for PSS. Currently, airway diseases, in particular COPD with pulmonary emphysema, are the most common cause of pleural gas effusion. [17]. This has been demonstrated by the results of several studies in which pulmonary emphysema was the main cause of PSS, found in 32.8% of cases in the series by Tanaka et al. [21]68% of the 505 cases of PSS studied by Weissberg et al. [17]77% of cases in the retrospective study by Ruppert et al. [22] and in 73.3% of cases in the series by Onuki et al. [19]. PS can occur during the course of COPD, mainly as a result of the rupture of subpleural emphysematous bullous zones favored by thoracic distension. [21]. Other airway diseases that can cause PS include asthma, cystic fibrosis and bronchiolitis obliterans. Asthma can be responsible for PS in the event of a severe attack caused by a major increase in alveolar pressure. This complication may occur in 1% to 5% of cases, depending on the series [53]. Infectious pathologies in general, and pulmonary tuberculosis in particular, remain among the most common causes of PS in endemic areas of this condition, such as India [38,39]. This complication affects around 0.6 to 1.4% of patients suffering from this infectious disease during their treatment period. PS occurs either as a result of intra-pleural rupture of cavitary lesions, or as a result of extension of the necrotizing infectious process to the visceral pleura. It is sometimes complicated by pleural empyema and persistent bronchopleural fistula. [15]. Pneumothorax may occur in the course of other pulmonary infections, such as abscessed pneumonia caused by necrotizing germs, due to the rupture of a parenchymal abscess within the pleural cavity [55]. In AIDS, the incidence of PSS is 450 times higher than in the non-HIV-infected population, occurring in 2% of patients. These patients often have emphysematous lesions in the form of bullous dystrophies in the lung apex and cortical regions. Pneumocystis carinii pneumonia is the most common infectious pulmonary complication of AIDS. It represents an additional risk factor for the development of PS. Indeed, this fungal infection leads to necrotizing lesions of the lung parenchyma, with the formation of apical and subpleural cystic cavities at the origin of PSS in 5 to 10% of cases [56]. SIDs are also a frequent cause of SP. Idiopathic pulmonary fibrosis (IPF) is one of the most common IDPs. In the course of this condition, an SBP affects one in 167 people each year, and is thought to be secondary to the rupture of subpleural honeycomb lesions [58-59]. PS may reveal Langerhansian Histiocytosis, which should be suspected in a male smoker with cystic lesions on chest CT [65] , or lymphangioleiomyomatosis in 42% of cases, which is a rare pathology in women of childbearing age [66] and less frequently pneumoconiosis and connectivites such as rheumatoid arthritis, scleroderma and ankylosing spondylitis [63, 64, 65]. Pneumothorax is rarer in mediastino-pulmonary sarcoidosis, described in 2% of cases, and occurs following rupture of a subpleural bulla or necrosis of a subpleural granuloma [65]. PS may also complicate malignant pulmonary pathologies, notably subcortical metastases and malignant pleural mesothelioma, but also primary bronchopulmonary cancer, which may be revealed by a gaseous pleural effusion in 0.03% and 0.05% of cases [66]. Pohl et al. estimated that 2% of PS are secondary to a malignant pulmonary pathology, whether primary or secondary[67]. Possible mechanisms of PS secondary to tumor pathology are [68] :

- Tumor wall necrosis with rupture into the pleural space.
- The presence of endobronchial lesions that act as a valve mechanism leading to the development and rupture of subpleural bullae.
- Presence of broncho-pleural fistula.

Other, rarer causes of pneumothorax include Marfan's disease, Birt-Hogg-Dube syndrome, etc. [69] and catamenial pneumothorax [70]. The latter occurs in young women on the eve of menstruation and 72 hours after its onset. The mechanism by which SP occurs remains controversial, and four theories have been put forward to explain its pathogenesis [71] :

- Spontaneous rupture of blebs.
- The existence of diaphragmatic pleural defects.
- Alveolar rupture due to bronchospasm and vasoconstriction induced by increased blood and local levels of prostaglandin F2 during menstruation
- And finally, the desquamation of pleural endometriosis which, during menstruation, can cause an air passage.

In our series, COPD with pulmonary emphysema topped the list of etiologies of PSS found in 71.6% of cases, in line with the literature, followed by bronchial dilatation sequelae of pulmonary tuberculosis in 10.8% of cases, then neoplastic causes in 6.6% of cases and fibrosing PID in 5.4% of cases. Active pulmonary tuberculosis was responsible for 4.1% of cases of PSS.

The role of the scanner in the therapeutic management of PS

Chest X-rays are the first-line examination for diagnosing a PS and guiding its immediate therapeutic management. Chest CT scans are reserved, according to the recommendations of learned societies, for recurrent pneumothorax, in cases of doubt as to the aberrant location of the chest tube, or in cases of prolonged air leakage lasting more than five to seven days. This examination is also indicated preoperatively to guide surgical treatment of PS and any associated procedures, such as biopsy specimens required to diagnose the causative pulmonary pathology, such as PID or lung volume reduction surgery [1,7,72]. However, the role and usefulness of chest CT in predicting the risk of PS recurrence remains controversial. In their study of 231 cases of PSP, Huang et al demonstrated that the factors associated with contralateral recurrence of PSP were low body weight (BMI<18.5 kg/m^2) and the presence of blebs on the contralateral lung as demonstrated by high-resolution CT scan [73]. The authors conclude that this group of patients could justify video-assisted thoracoscopy from the outset to prevent recurrence. In another prospective study, the authors found that contralateral recurrence of a first episode of PSP was statistically associated with the presence of bullae on that lung demonstrated by a preoperative chest CT scan of the first affected lung. According to the authors, it would therefore be legitimate to propose surgery to prevent early recurrence in these patients [74].

The first "bleb score" was proposed by Warner et al in 1991 [75]. The authors assigned a number from one to five for blebs according to their size (1 for a size of 0 to 5 mm, 2 from 6 to 10 mm, 3 from 11 to 21 mm, 4 from 21 to 30 mm and 5 over 31 mm). The score was obtained by multiplying the number of blebs in each category by its number. The score was significantly higher in subjects with recurrent pneumothorax requiring surgical pleurodesis. According to this study, chest CT could be useful in predicting the risk of PSP recurrence and defining patients warranting pleural symphysis from the outset. Numerous other studies support the systematic performance of a chest CT scan in the face of a first episode of PSP in order to define the risk of recurrence and to be able to propose a personalized preventive approach [65, 66].

Contrary to these data, other authors have found no correlation between bullous dystrophy on chest CT and the risk of recurrence of PS [67, 68]. In their prospective study involving 35 patients with PSP explored by thoracic CT, Mitlehner et al found no correlation between the risk of PS recurrence and the number, size and distribution of dystrophic lesions on thoracic CT [41]. These data are confirmed by the study by Smit et al, who found no statically significant relationship between the presence and location of bullous lesions on chest CT scans of 101 patients with PSP and the risk of pneumothorax recurrence [80]. In another prospective study involving 55 patients who underwent chest CT after resolution of the pneumothorax episode, the authors demonstrated the absence of an association between the presence, number, size and location of bullae on chest CT and the risk of recurrence of PS. The authors therefore did not recommend surgery for the resection of bullae after a first episode of PSP on the basis of the scannographic data [81]. In a Tunisian study carried out in 2007, Besbes et al evaluated the association between recurrence of PSP and the results of chest CT scans performed on 80 patients within one week of hospital discharge. [82]. The "dystrophic lesion" score was based on the same criteria used by Warner in 1991 [75]. Dystrophic bullae were present on CT in 72.5% of patients. The severity of these lesions deduced from the dystrophic score was not statistically associated with the risk of recurrence. The authors thus concluded that dystrophic bullous lesions are frequently present in PSP without being associated with an increased risk of recurrence.

Given the disparity of these results, the decision to perform pleurodesis based on the presence of blebs or bullae on CT is not justified at this time. [5, 8]. During the follow-up period of our study, 16 PS recurrences were observed. They were more frequent in PSS than in PSP (14.9% versus 3.8%; p=0.004). No statistically significant relationship was found between the presence of blebs or emphysema on chest CT, the location of these lesions, their type and pneumothorax recurrence. However, the relationship between the extent of emphysema and the risk of recurrence was not studied, as the analysis of emphysematous lesions was qualitative and not quantitative.

C ONCLUSIONS

Classification of PS as primary or secondary is based primarily on clinical and chest X-ray findings. A thoracic CT scan is only indicated in the event of persistent doubt about a parenchymal pathology not identified by these initial investigations. Outside this context, the role of this examination in the etiological investigation of a PS is not well codified. Its contribution to predicting the risk of recurrence, the main evolutionary risk of a PS, also remains a subject of controversy.

With the aim of determining the etiological profile of PS and identifying the role of CT scanning in the etiological investigation of this condition as well as in its therapeutic management, we conducted a prospective study of 206 cases of PS managed at the Pneumology Department of Mohamed Taher Mâamouri Hospital in Nabeul between August 2013 and December 2019. Determination of the primary or secondary nature of the PS was based on BTS criteria considering as PSS any PS occurring in a patient over 50 years of age with a history of heavy smoking or in a patient with clinical signs or chest X-ray abnormalities in favor of an underlying pulmonary pathology. In all other cases, PS is considered to be primary.

The mean age of our population was 40 ± 18 years [16-87]. A clear male predominance was noted, with a M/F gender ratio of 40.2. Most of our patients were active smokers (88.8%). Respiratory comorbidity was known at the time of PS diagnosis in 55 patients (26.7% of cases), with COPD in 36 (17.5%), asthma in four (2%), active pulmonary tuberculosis in three (1,4%) and cured with parenchymal sequelae in nine patients (4.3%), fibrosing IPD in two patients (1%) (one case of idiopathic pulmonary fibrosis and one case of mediastino-pulmonary sarcoidosis) and primary pulmonary neoplasia in one patient. Chest pain was the main clinical warning sign, reported by 183 patients (88.8% of cases), followed by dyspnea reported by 72 patients (35%). Chest X-rays, taken for all patients on admission, showed parenchymal abnormalities in favor of underlying pulmonary pathology in 50 cases (24.2%). These abnormalities were represented by pulmonary emphysema in 34 cases (16.5%), retractile opacity with areolar images suggestive of pulmonary tuberculosis sequelae in eight cases (3.8%), round intra-parenchymal opacities in six cases (2.9%) (single in three patients and multiple in three), cystic images in two patients (1%) and cavitary in one case (0.5%), and interstitial syndrome in four cases (1.9%). In our study, we identified 132 cases of PSP (64.1%) and 74 cases of PSS, based on clinical and chest X-ray data. Several studies have demonstrated the high prevalence of PSP compared with PSS. Patients with PSP were younger than those with PSS, with an average age of 29 ± 9 years versus 60.6 years ($p<0.001$), and more often had a lanky morphotype (27.3% versus 12.2%; $p=0.012$). It has been well demonstrated in the literature that PSP is a pathology of young subjects with a lanky morphotype, whereas PSS classically affects smokers over 50. Chest pain was more frequent in the PSP group than in the PSS group (96.2% versus 75.6%; $p<0.001$), while dyspnea was more frequently noted in the PSS group (45.9% versus 28.7%; $p=0.013$). Unlike PSP, PSS is often poorly tolerated from a respiratory standpoint, due to low ventilatory reserve secondary to underlying parenchymal pathology and the patient's generally more advanced age. Chest CT scans were performed on 93 patients in the PSP group (70.5%) and 70 patients in the PSS group (94.6%) ($p<0.001$). The indications for this examination were the assessment of underlying parenchymal lesions for 78 patients (55/93 patients in the PSP group (59.1%) and 23/70 patients in the PSS group (32.9%); $p=0.001$), recurrent pneumothorax for 17 patients (6/93 patients in the PSP group (6.5%) and 11/70 patients in the PSS group (15.7%); $p=0.055$), persistent pneumothorax in 36 patients (19/93 patients in the PSP group (20.4%) and 17 patients in the PSS group (24.3%); $p=0.55$), suspected complication of chest drainage in 23 patients (13/93 patients in the PSP group (14%) and 10/70 patients in the PSS group (14.3%); $p=0.9$) and doubt between partial pneumothorax and emphysema bulla in nine patients in the PSS group (12.9%). In the PSP group, chest CT revealed apical blebs in 16/93 cases (17.2%) and pulmonary emphysema lesions in 49 patients (52.7%). It would be legitimate to question the truly primitive nature of PS in these 49 cases. However, none of them showed signs of COPD during the follow-up period. In the PSS group, the thoracic CT scan provided a more accurate assessment of the etiology of PS, revealing abnormalities not detected by the thoracic X-ray in 44.3% of cases, such as pulmonary emphysema in all cases.

Several studies have demonstrated the superiority of CT scans for the assessment of underlying parenchymal lesions in PS. Increasingly, patients suffering from PSP are discovering abnormalities, notably emphysema lesions, which would have gone unnoticed on a simple chest X-ray. However, these lesions are not always synonymous with respiratory disease, and their clinical significance is not well established.

In our study, the etiologies considered for PSS were dominated by COPD with pulmonary emphysema (71.6% of PSS), followed by sequelae of pulmonary tuberculosis in 10.8% of cases. Active pulmonary tuberculosis accounted for 4.1% of PSS cases. COPD with pulmonary emphysema is the most common cause of pleural gas effusion, particularly in developed countries, ahead of infectious causes in general and pulmonary tuberculosis in particular, which continues to represent one of the main causes of PSS in areas with high tuberculosis endemicity.

Pleurodesis was performed in 48 patients. It was medical through the drain for 13 patients in the PSS group (6%) and surgical for 35 patients (17%) (19 patients in the PSP group (14.4%) and 16 patients in the PSS group (21.6%); p=0.3). A preoperative chest CT scan was performed in all cases. This examination revealed parenchymal abnormalities in 29 patients (13/19 patients in the PSP group (68.4%) and 16/16 patients in the PSS group (100%); p=0.02). These abnormalities were mainly blebs in 3/19 patients in the PSP group (15.8%) and pulmonary emphysema in 25 patients (10/19 patients in the PSP group (76.9%) and 15/16 patients in the PSS group (93.8%); p=0.29). The operative procedures associated with pleurodesis were bullae resection in 16/35 patients (45.7%), bleb resection in 1/35 patients (2.9%), cure of a pulmonary hydatid cyst in one patient (2.9%) and surgical lung biopsy in one patient. A thoracic CT scan is often indicated prior to surgery for a PS. It enables a precise lesion assessment to be established, and helps to guide the operative procedures associated with pleurodesis, such as a surgical lung biopsy required to diagnose an underlying PID.

In our study, recurrences were noted in 16 patients. They were more frequent in PSS than in PSP (14.9% versus 3.8% in PSS; p=0.004). There was no statistically significant relationship between the presence of blebs and the risk of recurrence, nor with the presence, location or type of emphysema. The relationship between the extent of pulmonary emphysema and the risk of recurrence could not be studied, as the analysis of emphysema lesions was qualitative and not quantitative.

Literature data on the usefulness of chest CT in predicting the risk of PS recurrence are contradictory. At present, apart from certain special situations such as bilateral pneumothorax and PS secondary to lymphangioleiomyomatosis, preventive pleurodesis cannot be proposed after a first episode of PS on the basis of CT findings alone.

At the end of this work, we can conclude that :

- Chest CT is superior to chest X-ray in assessing parenchymal lesions in PS. However, the clinical significance of these lesions is not well established. A systematic thoracic CT scan as part of the etiological assessment of PS does not therefore appear justified at present.
- Thoracic CT scans are systematically performed in cases of suspected underlying parenchymal pathology not elucidated by clinical and radiological data. In all other cases, its indication should be discussed on a case-by-case basis. It should be encouraged in all cases of PS in young women, as there is

a high probability of discovering an underlying parenchymal pathology such as lymphangioleiomyomatosis.

- Pulmonary emphysema is the most common abnormality associated with PSP. The discovery of such a lesion in patients initially classified as PSP should lead to prolonged clinical and respiratory functional follow-up, in order to detect the onset of COPD at an early stage.
- Scannographic data, in particular the presence of emphysema lesions, their location and type, cannot predict the risk of recurrence of PS in a given patient. Larger-scale prospective studies with qualitative as well as quantitative analysis of these lesions are needed to study the relationship between the extent of these lesions and the probability of pneumothorax recurrence, and to be able to propose a personalized preventive approach.

REF RENC ES

1. MacDuff A, Arnold A, Harvey J, on behalf of the BTS Pleural Disease Guideline Group. Management of spontaneous pneumothorax: British Thoracic Society pleural disease guideline 2010. Thorax. Aug 2010;65(Suppl 2):ii18-31.

2. Hallifax R, Janssen JP. Pneumothorax-Time for New Guidelines? Semin Respir Crit Care Med. Jun 2019;40(03):314-22.

3. Muramatsu T, Nishii T, Takeshita S, Ishimoto S, Morooka H, Shiono M. Preventing recurrence of spontaneous pneumothorax after thoracoscopic surgery: A review of recent results. Surg Today. Aug 2010;40(8):696-9.

4. Lippert HL, Lund O, Blegvad S, Larsen HV. Independent risk factors for cumulative recurrence rate after first spontaneous pneumothorax. Eur Respir J. Mar 1991;4(3):324-31.

5. Bintcliffe OJ, Hallifax RJ, Edey A, Feller-Kopman D, Lee YCG, Marquette CH, et al. Spontaneous pneumothorax: time to rethink management? Lancet Respir Med. Jul 2015;3(7):578-88.

6. Leyn PD, Lismonde M, Ninane V, Noppen M, Slabbynck H, Meerhaeghe AV, et al. Belgian Society of Pneumology. Guidelines on the management of spontaneous pneumothorax. Acta Chirurgica Belgica. Jan 2005;105(3):265-7.

7. Baumann MH, Strange C, Heffner JE, Light R, Kirby TJ, Klein J, et al. Management of spontaneous pneumothorax: an American College of Chest Physicians Delphi consensus statement. Chest. Feb 2001;119(2):590-602.

8. Grenier P. Imagerie thoracique de l'adulte. 3rd ed. Paris: Flammarion médecine-sciences; 2006.

9. Tschopp JM, Bintcliffe O, Astoul P, Canalis E, Driesen P, Janssen J, et al. ERS task force statement: diagnosis and treatment of primary spontaneous pneumothorax. Eur Respir J. Aug 2015;46(2):321-35.

10. Hansell DM, Bankier AA, MacMahon H, McLoud TC, Müller NL, Remy J. Fleischner Society: Glossary of Terms for Thoracic Imaging. Radiology. Mar 2008;246(3):697-722.

11. Ghisalberti M, Guerrera F, De Vico A, Bertolaccini L, De Palma A, Fiorelli A, et al. Age and Clinical Presentation for Primary Spontaneous Pneumothorax. Heart Lung Circ. Nov 2020;29(11):1648-55.

12. Bobbio A, Dechartres A, Bouam S, Damotte D, Rabbat A, Regnard JF, et al. Epidemiology of spontaneous pneumothorax: gender-related differences. Thorax. Jul 2015;70(7):653-8.

13. Porcel JM. Phenotyping primary spontaneous pneumothorax. Eur Respir J. Sept 2018;52(3):1801455.

14. Gupta D. Epidemiology of pneumothorax in England. Thorax. Aug 2000;55(8):666-71.

15. Huan NC, Sidhu C, Thomas R. Pneumothorax. Clinics in Chest Medicine. Dec 2021;42(4):711-27.

16. Ferraro P, Beauchamp G, Lord F, Emond C, Bastien E. Spontaneous primary and secondary pneumothorax: a 10-year study of management alternatives. Can J Surg. Jun 1994;37(3):197-202.

17. Weissberg D, Refaely Y. Pneumothorax. Chest. May 2000;117(5):1279-85.

18. Beji M, Pinet C, Gounant V, Gibelin A. Etiological factors. Rev Mal Respir Actual. Jun 2013;5(3):195-9.

19. Onuki T, Ueda S, Yamaoka M, Sekiya Y, Yamada H, Kawakami N, et al. Primary and Secondary Spontaneous Pneumothorax: Prevalence, Clinical Features, and In-Hospital Mortality. Can Respir J. Mar 2017;6014967.

20. Brown SGA, Ball EL, Macdonald SPJ, Wright C, McD Taylor D. Spontaneous pneumothorax; a multicentre retrospective analysis of emergency treatment, complications and outcomes: Spontaneous pneumothorax. Intern Med J. May 2014;44(5):450-7.

21. Tanaka F, Itoh M, Esaki H, Isobe J, Ueno Y, Inoue R. Secondary spontaneous pneumothorax. Ann. Cardiothorac. Surg. Feb 1993;55(2):372-6.

22. Ruppert AM, Sroussi D, Khallil A, Giot M, Assouad J, Cadranel J, et al. Detection of secondary causes of spontaneous pneumothorax: Comparison between computed tomography and chest X-ray. Diagn Interv Imaging. Apr 2020;101(4):217-24.

23. Hallifax RJ, Goldacre R, Landray MJ, Rahman NM, Goldacre MJ. Trends in the Incidence and Recurrence of Inpatient-Treated Spontaneous Pneumothorax, 1968-2016. JAMA. Oct 2018;320(14):1471-80.

24. Kim D, Jung B, Jang BH, Chung SH, Lee YJ, Ha IH. Epidemiology and medical service use for spontaneous pneumothorax: a 12-year study using nationwide cohort data in Korea. BMJ Open. Oct 2019;9(10):e028624.

25. Ruppert AM, Perrin J, Khalil A, Vieira T, Abou-Chedid D, Masmoudi H, et al. Effect of cannabis and tobacco on emphysema in patients with spontaneous pneumothorax. Diagn Interv Imaging. Aug 2018;99(7-8):465-71.

26. Saidi O, Malouche D, O'Flaherty M, Ben Mansour N, A Skhiri H, Ben Romdhane H, et al. Assessment of cardiovascular risk in Tunisia: applying the Framingham risk score to national survey data. BMJ Open. Nov 2016;6(11):e009195.

27. Hedevang Olesen W, Katballe N, Sindby JE, Titlestad IL, Andersen PE, Ekholm O, et al. Cannabis increased the risk of primary spontaneous pneumothorax in tobacco smokers: a case-control study. Eur J Cardiothorac Surg. Oct 2017;52(4):679-85.

28. Noppen M. Spontaneous pneumothorax: epidemiology, pathophysiology and cause. Eur Respir Rev. Sep 2010;19(117):217-9.

29. Lesur O, Delorme N, Polu JM, Fromaget JM, Bernadac P. Computed Tomography in the Etiologic Assessment of Idiopathic Spontaneous Pneumothorax. Chest. Aug 1990;98(2):341-7.

30. Massongo M, Leroy S, Scherpereel A, Vaniet F, Dhalluin X, Chahine B, et al. Outpatient management of primary spontaneous pneumothorax: a prospective study. Eur Respir J. Feb 2014;43(2):582-90.

31. Noppen M, Dekeukeleire T, Hanon S, Stratakos G, Amjadi K, Madsen P, et al. Fluorescein-enhanced Autofluorescence Thoracoscopy in Patients with Primary Spontaneous Pneumothorax and Normal Subjects. Am J Respir Crit Care Med. Jul 2006;174(1):26–30.

32. Chen CK, Chen PR, Huang HC, Lin YS, Fang HY. Overexpression of Matrix Metalloproteinases in Lung Tissue of Patients with Primary Spontaneous Pneumothorax. Respiration. 2014;88(5):418–25.

33. Maeda A, Ishioka S, Yoshihara M, Mihara M, Shigenobu T, Nakamura S. Primary Spontaneous Pneumothorax Detected During a Medical Checkup. Chest. Sep 1999;116(3):847–8.

34. Voge VM, Anthracite R. Spontaneous pneumothorax in the USAF aircrew population: a retrospective study. Aviat Space Environ Med. Oct 1986;57(10):939–49.

35. Abolnik IZ, Lossos IS, Gillis D, Breuer R. Primary Spontaneous Pneumothorax in Men. Am J Med Sci. May 1993;305(5):297–303.

36. Lauri H. High-resolution CT of the lungs: Indications and diagnosis. Duodecim. 2017;133(6):549–56.

37. Kang MJ, Park CM, Lee CH, Goo JM, Lee HJ. Dual-Energy CT: Clinical Applications in Various Pulmonary Diseases. RadioGraphics. May 2010;30(3):685–98.

38. Bense L, Lewander R, Eklund G, Hedenstierna G, Wiman LG. Nonsmoking, Non-Alpha1-Antitrypsin Deficiency-Induced Emphysema in Nonsmokers With Healed Spontaneous Pneumothorax, Identified by Computed Tomography of the Lungs. Chest. Feb 1993;103(2):433–8.

39. Bintcliffe OJ, Edey AJ, Armstrong L, Negus IS, Maskell NA. Lung Parenchymal Assessment in Primary and Secondary Pneumothorax. Annals ATS. Mar 2016;13(3):350–5.

40. Savitsky E, Oh SS, Lee JM. The Evolving Epidemiology and Management of Spontaneous Pneumothorax. JAMA. Oct 2018;320(14):1441.

41. Mitlehner W, Friedrich M, Dissmann W. Value of Computer Tomography in the Detection of Bullae and Blebs in Patients with Primary Spontaneous Pneumothorax. Respiration. 1992;59(4):221–7.

42. Kobayashi NS, Nambu A, Kawamoto M, Hayashi TY, Watanabe M, Okumura T, et al. Pulmonary Apical Opacities on Thin-Section Computed Tomography: Relationship to Primary Spontaneous Pneumothorax in Young Male Patients and Corresponding Histopathologic Findings. J Comput Assist Tomogr. 2018;42(1):33-8.

43. Lee KH, Kim KW, Kim EY, Lee JI, Kim YS, Hyun SY, et al. Detection of blebs and bullae in patients with primary spontaneous pneumothorax by multi-detector CT reconstruction using different slice thicknesses: Pneumothorax-different reconstruction methods in MDCT. J Med Imaging Radiat Oncol. Dec 2014;58(6):663-7.

44. Kim DH. The feasibility of axial and coronal combined imaging using multi-detector row computed tomography for the diagnosis and treatment of a primary spontaneous pneumothorax. J Cardiothorac Surg. May 2011;6(1):71.

45. Park C, Sung M, Lee G, Do Y, Park H, Kim J, et al. Risk of Primary Spontaneous Pneumothorax According to Chest Configuration. Thorac cardiovasc Surg. Oct 2018;66(07):583-8.

46. Epler GR, McLoud TC, Gaensler EA, Mikus JP, Carrington CB. Normal Chest Roentgenograms in Chronic Diffuse Infiltrative Lung Disease. N Engl J Med. Apr 1978;298(17):934-9.

47. Tsou KC, Huang PM, Hsu HH, Chen KC, Kuo SW, Lee JM, et al. Role of computed tomographic scanning prior to thoracoscopic surgery for primary spontaneous pneumothorax. J Formos Med Assoc. Sep 2014;113(9):606-11.

48. Hilliard NJ, Marciniak SJ, Babar JL, Balan A. Evaluation of secondary spontaneous pneumothorax with multidetector CT. Clin Radiol. May 2013;68(5):521-8.

49. Johannesma PC, Reinhard R, Kon Y, Sriram JD, Smit HJ, van Moorselaar RJA, et al. Prevalence of Birt-Hogg-Dubé syndrome in patients with apparently primary spontaneous pneumothorax. Eur Respir J. Apr 2015;45(4):1191-4.

50. Hagaman JT, Schauer DP, McCormack FX, Kinder BW. Screening for Lymphangioleiomyomatosis by High-Resolution Computed Tomography in Young, Nonsmoking Women Presenting with Spontaneous Pneumothorax Is Cost-Effective. Am J Respir Crit Care Med. Jun 2010;181(12):1376-82.

51. Gupta N, Finlay GA, Kotloff RM, Strange C, Wilson KC, Young LR, et al. Lymphangioleiomyomatosis Diagnosis and Management: High-Resolution Chest Computed Tomography, Transbronchial Lung Biopsy, and Pleural Disease Management. An Official American Thoracic Society/Japanese Respiratory Society Clinical Practice Guideline. Am J Respir Crit Care Med. Nov 2017;196(10):1337-48.

52. Davies HE, Wathen CG, Gleeson FV. The risks of radiation exposure related to diagnostic imaging and how to minimise them. BMJ. Feb 2011;342:d947.

53. O'Rourke JP, Yee ES. Civilian Spontaneous Pneumothorax. Chest. Dec 1989;96(6):1302-6.

54. Singh SK, Tiwari KK. Analysis of clinical and radiological features of tuberculosis associated pneumothorax. Indian J Tuberc. Jan 2019;66(1):34-8.

55. Tumbarello M, Tacconelli E, Pirronti T, Cauda R, Ortona L. Pneumothorax in HIV-infected patients: role of Pneumocystis carinii pneumonia and pulmonary tuberculosis. Eur Respir J. Jun 1997;10(6):1332-5.

56. Coker RJ, Moss F, Peters B, McCarty M, Nieman R, Claydon E, et al. Pneumothorax in patients with AIDS. Respir Med. Jan 1993;87(1):43-7.

57. Nishimoto K, Fujisawa T, Yoshimura K, Enomoto Y, Enomoto N, Nakamura Y, et al. The prognostic significance of pneumothorax in patients with idiopathic pulmonary fibrosis: Pneumothorax in patients with IPF. Respirology. May 2018;23(5):519-25.

58. Franquet T, Giménez A, Torrubia S, Sabaté JM, Rodriguez-Arias JM. Spontaneous pneumothorax and pneumomediastinum in IPF. Eur Radiol. Jan 2000;10(1):108-13.

59. Flume PA, Strange C, Ye X, Ebeling M, Hulsey T, Clark LL. Pneumothorax in Cystic Fibrosis. Chest. Aug 2005;128(2):720-8.

60. Suri HS, Yi ES, Nowakowski GS, Vassallo R. Pulmonary langerhans cell histiocytosis. Orphanet J Rare Dis. Dec 2012;7(1):16.

61. Excoffier S, Guinand O, Rochat T. Pulmonary lymphangioleimyomatosis: review and case report. Rev Med Suisse. Aug 2016;12(527):1390-3.

62. Bouros D, Pneumatikos I, Tzouvelekis A. Pleural Involvement in Systemic Autoimmune Disorders. Respiration. 2008;75(4):361-71.

63. Kaneda H, Saito Y, Okamoto M, Maniwa T, Minami K ichiro, Imamura H. Bilaterally repeated spontaneous pneumothorax with ankylosing spondylitis. Gen Thorac Cardiovasc Surg. Jun 2007;55(6):266-9.

64. Le Pavec J, Launay D, Mathai SC, Hassoun PM, Humbert M. Scleroderma Lung Disease. Clinic Rev Allerg Immunol. Apr 2011;40(2):104-16.

65. Manika K, Kioumis I, Zarogoulidis K, Kougioumtzi I, Dryllis G, Pitsiou G, et al. Pneumothorax in sarcoidosis. J Thorac Dis. Oct 2014;6(Suppl 4):S466-469.

66. Steinhäuslin CA, Cuttat JF. Spontaneous Pneumothorax. Chest. Nov 1985;88(5):709-13.

67. Pohl D, Herse B, Criée CP, Dalichau H. Spontaneous pneumothorax as the initial symptom of bronchial cancer. Pneumologie. Feb 1993;47(2):69-72.

68. Maniwa T, Nakagawa K, Isaka M, Ohde Y, Okumura T, Kondo H. Pneumothorax associated with treatment for pulmonary malignancy. Interact Cardiovasc Thorac Surg. Sep 2011;13(3):257-61.

69. Menko FH, van Steensel MA, Giraud S, Friis-Hansen L, Richard S, Ungari S, et al. Birt-Hogg-Dubé syndrome: diagnosis and management. Lancet Oncol. Dec 2009;10(12):1199-206.

70. Legras A, Alifano M. Thoracic endometriosis and catamenial pneumothorax. Rev Mal Respir. Sep 2011;28(7):852-3.

71. Anastasio C, Wémeau-Stervinou L, Jaillard S, Mariage P, Wallaert B. Catamenial pneumothorax: an often misunderstood diagnosis. Rev Pneumol Clin. Feb 2013;69(1):50–4.

72. Stanko S, Oesterle C, Lowe MC. High-Resolution CT Following Primary Spontaneous Pneumothorax in Adolescents: Useful Tool or Wasted Radiation? Cureus. May 2021;13(5):e14936.

73. Huang TW, Lee SC, Cheng YL, Tzao C, Hsu HH, Chang H, et al. Contralateral Recurrence of Primary Spontaneous Pneumothorax. Chest. Oct 2007;132(4):1146–50.

74. Sihoe ADL, Yim APC, Lee TW, Wan S, Yuen EHY, Wan IYP, et al. Can CT Scanning Be Used To Select Patients With Unilateral Primary Spontaneous Pneumothorax for Bilateral Surgery? Chest. Aug 2000;118(2):380–3.

75. Warner BW, Bailey WW, Shipley RT. Value of computed tomography of the lung in the management of primary spontaneous pneumothorax. Am J Surg. Jul 1991;162(1):39–42.

76. Olesen WH, Katballe N, Sindby JE, Titlestad IL, Andersen PE, Lindahl-Jacobsen R, et al. Surgical treatment versus conventional chest tube drainage in primary spontaneous pneumothorax: a randomized controlled trial. Eur J Cardiothorac Surg. Jul 2018;54(1):113–21.

77. Casali C, Stefani A, Ligabue G, Natali P, Aramini B, Torricelli P, et al. Role of Blebs and Bullae Detected by High-Resolution Computed Tomography and Recurrent Spontaneous Pneumothorax. Ann Cardiothorac Surg. Jan 2013;95(1):249–55.

78. Amjadi K, Alvarez GG, Vanderhelst E, Velkeniers B, Lam M, Noppen M. The Prevalence of Blebs or Bullae Among Young Healthy Adults. Chest. Oct 2007;132(4):1140–5.

79. Al-Githmi I. Is There a Role for Chest Computed Tomography in Patients with Primary Spontaneous Pneumothorax? Surg Sci. 2017;08(10):429–35.

80. Smit HJ, Wienk MA, Schreurs AJ, Schramel FM, Postmus PE. Do bullae indicate a predisposition to recurrent pneumothorax?Br J Radiol. Apr 2000;73(868):356–9.

81. Martínez-Ramos D, Ángel-Yepes V, Escrig-Sos J, Miralles-Tena JM, Salvador-Sanchís JL. Usefulness of Computed Tomography in Determining Risk of Recurrence After a First Episode of Primary Spontaneous Pneumothorax: Therapeutic Implications. Arch Bronconeumol. Jan 2007;43(6):304–8.

82. Ouanes-Besbes L, Golli M, Knani J, Dachraoui F, Nciri N, El Atrous S, et al. Prediction of recurrent spontaneous pneumothorax: CT scan findings versus management features. Respir Med. Feb 2007;101(2):230–6.

APPENDICES

Appendix 1:

Data collection form

DM: .... Entered on: ....../....../...... Released on: ....../......./.......
Number of hospital days: .... jrs
Admission through: ▪ Emergency ▪ SAMU ▪ C.E Pneumo ▪ Transfer from another department: ....
Last name: .... First name: .... Age: ....
Gender: ▪ Male ▪ Female
Place of residence: .... Origin: ▪ Urban ▪ Rural
School level: ....Profession:..............................
▪ Scuba diving ▪ Piloting
Active smoking: ▪ Yes .... PA ▪ No ▪Cannabis
Weaned: ▪ Yes since ......y ▪ Currently weaning (< 1y) ▪ No
ATCDs: ▪ COPD ▪ Asthma ▪ Pulmonary tuberculosis ▪ DDB ▪ KBP
▪ IRC ▪ PID ▪ Other ....
▪ PNO: ▪ right ▪ left ▪ bilateral
▪ Total ▪ Partial
▪ Old chest x-ray: ▪ Yes ▪ No
If yes :
▪ Distance apex - cupola = ... cm
▪ Interpleural distance at hilum height = ... cm
▪ Mediastinal bypass
▪ Bubbles ▪ Emphysema
▪ Pleuresis
▪ Other lung and pleural lesions: ....
▪▪1er episode .... months ago, treated with : ▪ simple monitoring
▪ Exsufflation
▪ Chest drainage

▪▪2ème episode .... months ago, treated with: ▪ simple monitoring ▪ exsufflation ▪ chest drainage

▪▪3ème episode .... months ago, treated with: ▪ simple monitoring ▪ exsufflation ▪ chest drainage
▪ hypertension ▪ coronary heart disease ▪ heart valve disease ▪ diabetes ▪ arterial disease
▪ Dyslipidemia ▪ HIV other: ....
Weight: .... kg Height: .... cm BMI: ....kg/m2 SC: m2
Morphotype: ▪ Normal ▪ Longline ▪ Marfan

PNO :
▪ Trauma: ....
▪ Iatrogenic
▪ Spontaneous: ▪ Idiopathic ▪ Secondary (type of respiratory pathology): ....
▪ Right ▪ Left ▪ Bilateral
▪ Total ▪ Partial

• 1st episode • (......) recurrence: • homolateral • contralateral
Occurrence during menstruation: • Yes • No
Time between onset of symptoms and consultation: .... days

CIRCUMSTANCES OF DISCOVERY

• Incidental discovery
• Chest pain: evolution over the past .... hours (or .... days) EVA: ..../10
• Rest dyspnea
• Exertional dyspnea Intensity: ....
• General signs: ....

Clinical examination:

• RR : ..../mn SpO2 = ...% BP : ... mmHg Pulse : ....../mn Other : ......
• Stable EHD (RR ≤ 24 c/min, SpO2 (AA) > 90%, 60 ≤ HR < 120, BP correct, patient can respond with whole sentences between breaths)
• EHD unstable
• Suffocating PNO
• Weight: ....Size: ....IMC: ....
• Other clinical signs: ....

GDS (AA): pH = ... PaO2 = ... mmHg PaCO2 = ...mmHg HCO3- = ...mmol/l Sat O2 = ...%

Chest x-ray:

• PNO partial • PNO total
• Distance apex - cupola = ... cm
• Interpleural distance at hilum height = ... cm
• Mediastinal bypass
• Bubbles • Subcutaneous emphysema • Pneumomediastinum • Abundant pleurisy..................
• Other lesions: ....

Chest CT scan: **Date: ....**

• Not done • Done, within .... days of positive diagnosis of PNO
• Normal
• Blebs: headquarters: ....
•Emphysème ....
• DDB • PID
• Other lesions: ....

Processing :

• Rest
• O2 Flow = ... l/mn
• Exsufflation Needle diameter = ... mm
• Pleurocatheter Catheter diameter = ... mm
• Heimlich valve • Pleurevac • Water jar

About drainage :

• Drain diameter: ....
• Diameter of drainage point = ... mm
• Drainage point location: ....

· Introduced drain length: ....
· Aspiration: · Immediate · Delayed: Time to drainage: ......
· Clamping test · Clamping time = ... hours
· Number of drainage days: .... days
·Optimisation background treatment: ....
Air is evacuated from the pleural cavity by :
· A pulmonologist · A pulmonology resident · A surgeon · A surgical resident
· A surgical resident · Other: ....
Air exhaust location :
· Pneumology · Emergency · Surgery
· Resuscitation department · Other department: ....
Evacuation carried out: · Matin· Afternoon · Evening
· Immediate success: · Lung to wall · Interpleural distance < 2 cm
· Success in less than 7 days (specify time): ....
· Detachment persistence > 48h
Complications :
· Bleeding · low abundance · medium abundance · high abundance
· OAP in vacuo
· Atelectasis
· Drainage site infection
· Purulent pleurisy
· Hemothorax: cc
· Subcutaneous drain path
· Subcutaneous emphysema Extent: ....
· Need to redo drain: cause ....
· Need to remove the drain because it is too far in
· Hospital stay = ... days
· Rx after drain removal: ....
Surgical treatment Date: ....
· Indication
· PNO persistent
· PNO toggle
· Recurrent PNO Number of recurrences = ...
· Bilateral PNO · Hemopneumothorax
· Other: ....

Type of pleurodesis
· Pleural abrasion · Partial pleurectomy · Other: ....
· Intraoperative talcation · Electrocoagulation · Intraoperative betadine · Talc through the drain
· Betadine through drain Protocol: ....
Treatment of underlying pulmonary lesions
· Bubble resection
· Bleb resection · Other: ....
Board of Directors

- Air travel banned for a month
- Lifetime diving ban
- Explanation of the risk of recidivism
- Tips for quitting smoking
- Reconsult in case of dyspnea

Time to return to work: .... days
Long-term trends

<u>- Consultation</u> (1): Date: ....
- Recurrence Delay: .... (Weeks)
- Physical examination: • RR: ..../mn SpO2 = ...% BP: ... mmHg Pulse: ....../mn Other: ....
- Homolateral seat • Contralateral seat.
- Chest pain EVA: ....
- Unsightly scar Appearance........... Diameter..........cm
- Smoking cessation (specify delay/pneumothorax): ....
- Passive smoking

Chest X-ray: ....

<u>- Consultation</u> (2): Date: ....
- Physical examination: • RR: ..../mn SpO2 = ...% BP: ... mmHg Pulse: ....../mn Other: ....
- Recurrence Delay: .... (Weeks)
- Homolateral location • Contralateral location
- Chest pain EVA: ....
- Unsightly scar
- Smoking cessation (specify delay/pneumothorax): ....
- Passive smoking

Chest X-ray...

<u>- Consultation</u> (3): Date:..............................
- Physical examination: • RR: ..../mn SpO2 = ...% BP: ... mmHg Pulse: ....../mn Other: ....
- Recidivism

Delay: .... (Weeks)
- Homolateral location • Contralateral location
- Chest pain EVA :...
- Unsightly scar
- Smoking cessation (specify delay/pneumothorax): ....
- Passive smoking

Chest X-ray: ....

ETIOLOGY OF SPONTANEOUS PNEUMOTHORAX: A 206-CASE STUDY

Abstract

Backround:

The etiological investigation of spontaneous pneumothorax (SP) is not standardized and the place of chest CT in this indication remains controversial.

The aim of our study was to determine the etiological profile of SP and to identify the role of chest CT in determining the etiology of this disease as well as in its therapeutic management.

Methods:

Prospective and descriptive study involving patients hospitalized for SP at the pneumology department of Mohamed Taher Mâamouri Hospital in Nabeul between August 2013 and December 2019.

Results:

Our study included 206 patients with a mean age of 40 ± 18 years. Respiratory comorbidity was already known in 55 patients (26.7%). Abnormalities in favour of an underlying pulmonary pathology were noted on the chest X-ray in 50 cases (24.2%). SP was classified as primary spontaneous pneumothorax (PSP) in 132 of cases (64.1%) and as secondary spontaneous pneumothorax in 74 of cases (SSP) (35.9%). In the PSP group, chest CT scans were performed in 93 patients (70.4%) and showed infra-radiological abnormalities such as pulmonary emphysema in 52.7% of cases. None of these patients showed signs of chronic obstructive pulmonary disease (COPD). In the SSP group, the CT scan performed on 70 patients (94.6%) identified abnormalities not visualized on the chest X-ray such as blebs or emphysema in 44.3% of cases. Chronic obstructive pulmonary disease with pulmonary emphysema topped the list of etiologies for SSP (71.6%), followed by bronchiectasis as sequelae of pulmonary tuberculosis (10.8%) and neoplastic diseases (6.6%). Recurrence of pneumothorax was more frequent in the SSP group than in the PSP group (p=0.004). No correlation was found between the presence of blebs or emphysema lesions, their location and type on chest CT scan and the risk of recurrence.

Conclusion:

Emphysema is the most common lesion for MS. CT is superior to chest X-ray in detecting this abnormality. The contribution of CT in determining the risk of recurrence of MS has not yet been established.

Key-words: Spontaneous pneumothorax, Etiologies, Chest CT

ETIOLOGICAL PROFILE OF SPONTANEOUS PNEUMOTHORAX IN 206 CASES

Summary

Introduction :

The etiological investigation of spontaneous pneumothorax (SP) is not standardized, and the role of chest CT in this indication remains controversial.

The aim of our study was to determine the etiological profile of PS and to identify the role of chest CT in determining the etiologies of this condition, as well as in its therapeutic management.

Methods :

Prospective and descriptive study involving patients hospitalized for PS at the Pneumology Department of Mohamed Taher Mâamouri Hospital in Nabeul between August 2013 and December 2019.

Results :

Our study included 206 patients with a mean age of 40 ± 18 years. Respiratory comorbidity was already known in 55 patients (26.7%). Abnormalities in favor of an underlying pulmonary pathology were noted on chest X-ray in 50 cases (24.2%). PS was classified as primary spontaneous pneumothorax (PSP) in 132 cases (64.1%) and secondary spontaneous pneumothorax (PSS) in 74 cases (35.9%). In the PSP group, chest CT scans were performed in 93 patients (70.4%) and revealed infra-radiological abnormalities such as pulmonary emphysema in 52.7% of cases. None of these patients showed signs of chronic obstructive pulmonary disease. In the PSS group, CT scans performed on 70 patients (94.6%) identified abnormalities not visualized on chest X-ray, such as blebs or emphysema in 44.3% of cases. Chronic obstructive pulmonary disease with pulmonary emphysema topped the list of PSS etiologies (71.6%), followed by bronchial dilatation sequelae of pulmonary tuberculosis (10.8%) and neoplastic causes (6.6%). Pneumothorax recurrence was more frequent in the PSS group than in the PSP group ($p=0.004$). No significant association was found between the presence of blebs or emphysema lesions, their location and type on chest CT and the risk of recurrence.

Conclusion:

Emphysema is the most common lesion to cause PS. CT is superior to chest radiography in detecting this anomaly. The contribution of CT to determining the risk of recurrence of PS has not yet been established.

Key words: Spontaneous pneumothorax, Etiologies, Chest CT scan

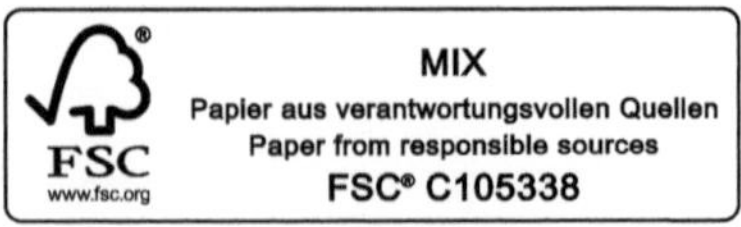

Printed by Books on Demand GmbH, Norderstedt / Germany